Power of Hormones: Your Guide to Optimal Hormone Health

A. Byrne

Contents

Introduction

Before we get down to business, I wanted to tell you a little about me and why I wrote this book!

I am 34 years old and married with three children who can be the most amazing little creatures - and the most horrific little monsters depending on the day!

I graduated from university with an honours degree in Psychology, and after two amazing years travelling overseas I decided it was time to settle down and find a job.

After a brief return to university to complete a graduate diploma in Human Resource Management, I started to carve out a career in Human Resources.

My husband and I got married, bought our first house and were looking forward to the rest of our lives. Little did we know that we were going to struggle to have children because of a condition I had.

I had suffered from heavy periods as a teenager, but didn't think much of it. My doctor told me, "It's normal and you need to get used to it."

So I did my best to get on with life. I have always been pretty active, I played a lot of sport, walked our high energy dog and loved going to gym classes - but I never seemed to lose any weight.

A visit to a new doctor revealed that I had polycystic ovarian syndrome. I was given a script for Metformin told to adhere to a Low GI diet and was sent on my way.

I didn't lose any weight and my symptoms didn't improve, but I was told there was nothing more they could do. I just needed to eat less and move more.

Some years later, we decided it was the right time to have children. However, we suffered months of bitter disappointed and negative pregnancy tests.

A visit to the gynaecologist and 3 laparoscopies later, I was diagnosed with stage III endometriosis. I was told that it was unlikely that I would fall pregnant naturally and we needed to book an appointment to discuss fertility assistance.

Of course, with the pressure now off, I fell pregnant naturally with a positive test result appearing the night before our first fertility appointment!

I wasn't one of those glowing pregnant women who loved being pregnant! I had a couple of small haemorrhages during the first trimester, and at 18 weeks pregnant I had an ovarian cyst rupture.

A ruptured cyst is horrendously painful when you're not pregnant, but the pain when you are pregnant is out of this world.

I ended up in hospital on a morphine pump. All throughout, I was plagued with guilt from thinking that I was hurting my baby with all these drugs in my system.

I developed pre-eclampsia at 34 weeks and went into pre-term labour at 35 weeks. I was told that if I wanted any more children, I would need to have them close together and that's exactly what we did!

In less than three years, it went from being just the two of us to five!

I was surprised (okay, I was over the moon!) to discover that I was losing weight rapidly after my third child! This had never happened before and it was amazing! Then, I stopped sleeping and I just didn't feel right.

I discovered that I had postpartum thyroiditis and was in a hyperthyroid state. The doctor told me not to worry. I would soon be hypothyroid and would eventually go back to normal in a couple of months.

He was right, the weight crept back on and life was back to normal - except for the huge growth on the side of my neck and this constant tiredness. I felt like the incredible hulk with this huge thick neck!

The thyroiditis had left a goiter in my neck and it just wouldn't go away. They decided to remove it, it was starting to press on my windpipe, so they removed the right lobe of my thyroid.

I had been kind of hoping that the surgery would have improved my fatigue, but sadly that wasn't the case. Every time I complained of being tired to a doctor, I would be brushed off and asked what did I expect with three young children.

I was made to feel like a drama queen and hypochondriac.

About 2 years later, the endometriosis came back in full force and I made the decision to have a hysterectomy. My gynaecologist recommended that I remove my uterus, but keep the ovaries so I didn't go into early menopause.

After the surgery, the surgeon visited me in recovery and told me that my uterus was a mess and it had looked as if it had been 'shredded'.

I had assumed that with all my problem bits now gone, my hormone issues would be over. I couldn't have been more wrong if I had tried!

Over the following 18 months, I visited a variety of general practitioners, naturopaths, endocrinologists and psychiatrists and was diagnosed with a series of conditions like chronic fatigue, and depression. I was prescribed so many different types of anti-depressants and stimulants, yet none of them worked.

I hated how many drugs I was putting into my body and I still felt sick. So I got rid of them all, flushed them down the toilet, and started to read everything I could on endocrine disorders.

It seemed logical to start with the thyroid, seeing as I knew mine played up every now and then. I discovered that if you have thyroid antibodies and a diagnosis of Hashimoto's, it is wise to treat it with Natural Desiccated Thyroid.

I was so excited! Imagine finally being able to get rid of that type of tiredness where all your bones feel like they're filled with concrete!

I went to the doctor and asked for a trial of NDT. She promptly told me that she never prescribes it as its unstable. My thyroid blood levels were within normal range, so I didn't need any treatment.

I was devastated - if I wasn't depressed before, I was starting to go that way now! I went back to the internet and learnt that holistic doctors were more likely to prescribe NDT.

I must have visited 6 doctors before stumbling across my amazing holistic doctor. The problem was that we lived at opposite ends of the country, but she told me she was happy to do Skype appointments.

She was willing to prescribe NDT, but wanted to see what all my other hormones were doing. This was the first time anybody had done this and I was intrigued to discover what they would reveal.

What we found was adrenal fatigue, estrogen dominance and Hashimoto's. A cocktail of badness and the reason for my fatigue, emotional fragility, hair loss, weight gain, acne and so much more.

This is when I started on my journey to wellness.

So why did I write this book? Well, I hate how long and difficult my journey has been and I wanted to make it easier for you.

This book is all my research around each of the conditions and symptoms.

It is a guide for you to use when making decisions on how to treat your conditions and even what tests you need to get them diagnosed.

I want you to become an expert on your health because nobody knows your body better than you. Let's find your optimal health and create hormonal harmony!

Chapter One:
The Vital Importance of Hormones

"Courage is the most important of all the virtues because without courage, you can't practice any other virtue consistently."
- Maya Angelou

- Our endocrine system is made up of 9 glands
- We produce hormones in each of these glands
- Hormones are needed for our most basic and our complex systems

What are Hormones?

Before we start delving into hormonal imbalances, it is important that we take a step back and look at the big picture! What are these pesky hormones and how do they all fit together?

The simplest way to explain what hormones are is to imagine them as little chemical messengers that are created in our endocrine glands. Their job is to travel through our bloodstream and send messages to other cells.

The types of messages they are delivering control many of our most basic functions. This includes hunger to our more intricate and delicate systems like reproduction, as well as our emotions and moods.

Our Endocrine System

When we talk about the endocrine system, we are simply talking about the hormone producing glands we have in our body. Specifically, we are talking about:

Hypothalamus: This gland controls the release of hormones from other glands as well as being responsible for our body temperature, hunger, moods, thirst, sleep and sex drive.

Parathyroid: These are our calcium controlling glands.

Thymus: This glands plays an important role for our immune system.

Pancreas: This is the insulin producing gland which helps control blood sugar levels.

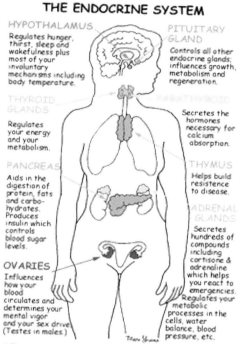

THE ENDOCRINE SYSTEM

HYPOTHALAMUS
Regulates hunger, thirst, sleep and wakefulness plus most of your involuntary mechanisms including body temperature.

PITUITARY GLAND
Controls all other endocrine glands; influences growth, metabolism and regeneration.

THYROID GLANDS
Regulates your energy and your metabolism.

PARATHYROID
Secretes the hormones necessary for calcium absorption.

PANCREAS
Aids in the digestion of protein, fats and carbo-hydrates. Produces insulin which controls blood sugar levels.

THYMUS
Helps build resistance to disease.

OVARIES
Influences how your blood circulates and determines your mental vigor and your sex drive. (Testes in males)

ADRENAL GLANDS
Secretes hundreds of compounds including cortisone & adrenaline which helps you react to emergencies. Regulates your metabolic processes in the cells, water balance, blood pressure, etc.

METABOLISM - The conversion of nutrients into energy and building materials to meet your body's needs.

Thyroid: The butterfly shaped gland produces thyroid hormones that control our metabolic rate and heart rate.

Adrenal: The adrenals are responsible for our fight or flight response, they control our sex drive and our stress hormone cortisol.

Pituitary: This gland is often called the "master control gland" and its job is to control all other glands as well as making sure we produce growth hormones.

Pineal: The pineal is responsible for producing serotonin derivatives of melatonin which becomes important when we start talking about sleep.

Ovaries: The ovaries are responsible for the production of estrogen, testosterone and progesterone in women.

Testes: The testes are responsible for the production of the male sex hormone, testosterone, in men.

This intricate system of glands manage our body's hormones and have a significant impact on our daily life. An imbalance in any of these areas can cause significant disruptions to our health and well being.

Hormones

Before we go any further, it is important for you to understand what are our major hormones and what do they do.

The chart below gives you an overview of most of the hormones in our body. We are going to focus on the hormones that frequently cause problems for women after puberty. These hormones are highlighted in yellow.

Gland	Hormone	Chemical Class	Actions	Regulated By
Hypothalamus				
Posterior Pituitary Gland	Oxytocin	Peptide	Stimulates contraction of uterus and mammary gland cells	Nervous system
	Antidiuretic hormone (ADH)	Peptide	Promotes retention of water by kidneys	Water/salt balance

Gland	Hormone	Chemical Class	Actions	Regulated By
Anterior Pituitary Gland	Growth hormone (GH)	Protein	Stimulates growth and metabolic functions	Hypothalamic hormones
	Prolactin (PRL)	Protein	Stimulates milk production and stimulation	Hypothalamic hormones
	Follicle-stimulating hormone (FSH)	Glyco-protein	Stimulates production of ova and sperm	Hypothalamic hormones
	Luteinizing hormone (LH)	Glyco-protein	Stimulates ovaries and testes	Hypothalamic hormones
	Thyroid-stimulating hormone (TSH)	Glyco-protein	Stimulates thyroid gland	Hypothalamic hormones
	Adrenocorticotropic hormone (ACTH)	Peptide	Stimulates adrenal cortex to secret glucocorticoids	Hypothalamic hormones
Thyroid Gland	Triiodothyronine (T3) Thyroxine (T4)	Amine	Stimulate and maintain metabolic processes	TSH
	Calcitonin	Peptide	Lowers blood calcium	Calcium in blood
Parathyroid Glands	Parathyroid hormone (PTH)	Peptide	Raises blood calcium	Calcium in blood
Pancreas	Insulin	Protein	Lowers blood glucose	Glucose in blood
	Glucagon	Protein	Raises blood glucose	Glucose in blood

Gland	Hormone	Chemical Class	Actions	Regulated By
Adrenal glands	Epinephrine Norepinephrine	Amines	Raise blood glucose, increase metabolic activities, constrict certain blood vessels	Nervous system
	Glucocorticoids	Steroid	Raise blood glucose	ACTH
	Mineralocorticoids	Steroid	Promote reabsorption of sodium and production of potassium in kidneys	Potassium in blood
Gonads	Androgens	Steroid	Support sperm formation and develop/maintain male secondary sex characteristics	FSH and LH
	Estrogens	Steroid	Stimulate uterine lining growth, promote development of female secondary sex characteristics	FSH and LH
	Progestins	Steroid	Promote uterine lining growth	FSH and LH
Pineal Gland	Melatonin	Amine	Involved in biological rhythms	Light/dark cycles

Before we get into the glands that cause the most problems - thyroid, adrenal, and ovaries – it's only fair to give you a quick summary of the glands we won't be examining in this book. They are important but don't quite cause the same chaos for women!

Posterior Pituitary Gland

The pituitary gland has two parts, the anterior and posterior. The anterior part is made up of gland cells and is connected to the brain by short blood vessels.

The posterior part is considered to be an actual part of the brain and it releases hormones straight into the bloodstream when told to by the brain.

The posterior part of the pituitary glands is responsible for the release of antidiuretic hormones which regulates the balance of water in our bodies. It also produces oxytocin which tells the uterus to contract when she is having a baby and tells the breasts to start releasing milk.

Parathyroid Glands

Strangely enough, the parathyroid glands are not related to the thyroid gland other than the fact they are attached to the thyroid gland. There are four of them and are located in your neck behind the thyroid.

They release parathyroid hormones, which regulate the level of calcium in our bodies with the help of calcitonin, which is produce and released by the thyroid.

Pancreas Basics

The pancreas produces insulin and glucagon to maintain a steady level of glucose in the body so that it has the fuel it needs to produce and maintain stores of energy. The condition most commonly associated with the pancreas is Diabetes.

There are two types of Diabetes - Type 1 is present from birth and Type 2 develops as you get older. Type 1 Diabetes is where the pancreas doesn't produce enough insulin causing blood sugar levels to drop. Type 2 Diabetes is when the body can't respond to insulin normally.

Pineal Gland

The pineal is in the middle of the brain and it secretes melatonin which is a very handy hormone that tells you to sleep at night and to wake up in the morning. The pineal gland uses the light and dark to determine when to release melatonin.

Chapter Two:
The Thyroid Puzzle

"I am old, Gandalf. I don't look it, but I am beginning to feel it my heart of hearts. Well-preserved indeed! Why, I feel all thin, sort of stretched, if you know what I mean: like butter that has been scraped over too much bread. That can't be right. I need a change, or something."
– Bilbo Baggins, "The Lord of the Rings: The Fellowship of the Ring"

- If you have a slow metabolism it could be a problem with your thyroid
- Your body makes 4 x as much T4 than T3
- Fatigue is a symptom of both hypothyroidism and hyperthyroidism
- Hypothyroid – too few thyroid hormones
- Hyperthyroid – too many thyroid hormones

Thyroid Basics

The thyroid gland is butterfly shaped gland located low in your neck. If your thyroid is 'normal', then you shouldn't be able to feel it.

The thyroids job is to regulate your metabolism. Your metabolism is responsible for making sure your body is able to break down food and convert it into energy.

Your thyroid controls the rate in which this process happens. A slower metabolism means your body may not be able to break down all the food you eat in a day and convert it to energy – it stores it as fat instead.

Hence the weight gain or the struggle to lose weight.

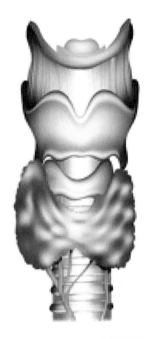
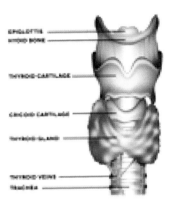

THYROID GLAND

Now, the hormones that we are going to refer to within this chapter are Thyroxine (T4) and Triiodothyronine (T3) – these are what people refer to as 'thyroid hormones'.

It's important to know that these hormones are not produced in equal numbers. We make about four times more T4 than T3. Once your thyroid gland has made these two hormones, they need to be released into your bloodstream.

The thyroid gland will only release your T3 and T4 hormones once it receives a message from your brain (pituitary gland) via a hormone known as a Thyroid Releasing Hormone (TRH).

Our bodies are clever and when functioning correctly our hormones are made to a strict recipe that suits our body and keep us balanced. When our body makes too much or too little of one of these hormones, this creates a hormonal imbalance and a series of symptoms that can affect our quality of life.

When talking about thyroid imbalances, you are considered to be **hypothyroid** if you have too little of the thyroid hormones. Having too many thyroid hormones is considered **hyperthyroid.**

Thyroid Symptoms

The table below is a list of common symptoms in hypothyroid or hyperthyroid patients.

If you believe you have 5 or more of the symptoms on either the hypothyroid or hyperthyroid list, it is very suggestive that your thyroid isn't functioning as it should. If you have 3-4 symptoms on the list, it is still likely that your thyroid could be the cause.

If it's less than 3, then we can't rule it out and it needs further investigation.

Hypothyroid (underactive)	Hyperthyroid (overactive)
Hair loss including outer 3rd of eyebrows	Fatigue
Dry skin/hair	Muscle weakness
Brittle fingernails	Hand tremors
Weight gain/difficulty losing weight	Mood swings
High cholesterol	Nervousness
Constipation	Anxiety

Hypothyroid (underactive)	Hyperthyroid (overactive)
Headaches	Rapid heartbeat – tachycardia
Decreased sweating	Dry skin
Muscle/joint aches	Difficulty sleeping
Tingling in hands/feet	Weight loss
Cold or hot intolerance	Diarrhoea
Slow speech	Light periods or missed periods
Slow heart rate	Heart palpitations
Fatigue	Hungrier than normal
Inability to concentrate	Sweating
Sluggish reflexes	Sensitive to the heat
Low sex drive	Dizziness
Heavy periods	Vision Changes
Infertility	
Depression or moody	

Hypothyroid Overview

- The most common cause of hypothyroidism is an autoimmune disease called Hashimoto's
- Is it your thyroid, pituitary or hypothalamus gland making you sick?
- Natural Desiccated Thyroid has been around since the 1950's

If you suspect you might be hypothyroid, you're probably feeling absolutely exhausted. Reading this book is hard work as you just can't seem to concentrate and feel like you must have ADHD!

You are also probably sick of cleaning out the waste trap in the bottom of your shower as your hair will be clogging it up. Your libido has probably disappeared and you are fed up with trying to lose weight.

All of this is more than likely leaving you feeling a bit low. If you were to describe your symptoms to a doctor, they may have suggested antidepressants and a bit of exercise.

It is incredibly frustrating being hypothyroid! By the end of this chapter, we will have had a look at why you might be hypothyroid, how you get diagnosed and most importantly, how to feel well again!

Causes/Conditions of Thyroid Dysfunction

The most common cause of hypothyroidism is **Hashimoto's Disease**. The name of this disease is pretty strange and it doesn't really give you any clues as to what it is!

Essentially, Hashimoto's Disease is an autoimmune disorder that causes your immune system to produce antibodies that attack your thyroid gland. It often causes thyroiditis which is a fancy term for inflammation of your thyroid gland.

These antibodies affect our thyroid glands ability to do its job of creating enough hormones.

Hashimoto's Disease is an example of **Primary Hypothyroidism,** when the problem is caused by the actual thyroid gland. Other less common causes of Primary Hypothyroidism are:

Thyroid Surgery – if you have a portion of your thyroid removed due to a goiter or growth, this may stop your thyroid functioning altogether. Also, it may not be able to perform as well as it did before the surgery.

Radiation Therapy – in some cancer patients, the radiation treatment they received in the neck area compromises their thyroid function as the radiation damages the cells within the thyroid.

Hyperthyroid Treatments – anti-thyroid medications and radioactive iodine are used to treat people with hyperthyroidism and occasionally these treatments can cause hypothyroidism by reducing the thyroid function.

Medications – Some drugs can affect the performance of your thyroid gland. For example, some heart, psychiatric and cancer treatments are known to interfere with the production of thyroid hormones. It is a good idea to check all your medications with your pharmacist and doctor to make sure that they will not affect the functioning of your thyroid gland.

Pregnancy – After the birth of my third child, I developed postpartum thyroiditis. My thyroid suddenly became inflamed, and it caused my thyroid hormone levels to increase into a hyperthyroid state and then suddenly drop back to hypothyroid levels. In most cases, the levels then return to their normal pre-pregnancy state within 6-12 months of delivery.

Congenital – Some babies are born with a thyroid that doesn't function correctly. There is no known reason why a baby's thyroid gland would not develop normally during pregnancy - particularly if there is no family history of thyroid disease.

Iodine Deficiency – Iodine in an important trace mineral that the thyroid gland needs to produce thyroid hormones. Where I live in New Zealand, we have a known iodine deficiency. The United States however, has nearly eliminated this problem. It is also important to note that too much iodine is also a problem! I have included a map on the next page for you to see if your country has an iodine deficiency.

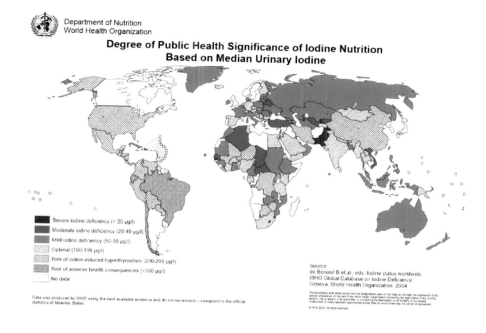

**Degree of Public Health Significance of Iodine Nutrition
Based on Median Urinary Iodine**

Severe iodine deficiency (< 20 µg/l)
Moderate iodine deficiency (20-49 µg/l)
Mild iodine deficiency (50-99 µg/l)
Optimal (100-199 µg/l)
Risk of iodine-induced hyperthyroidism (200-299 µg/l)
Risk of adverse health consequences (>300 µg/l)
No data

Source:
de Benoist B et al., eds. Iodine status worldwide.
WHO Global Database on Iodine Deficiency.
Geneva, World Health Organization, 2004.

Data was produced by WHO using the best available evidence and do not necessarily correspond to the official statistics of Member States

Secondary Hypothyroidism (or Central Hypothyroidism) - is
when the thyroid gland isn't the reason your thyroid gland isn't
producing enough thyroid hormones. Rather, it's caused by glands such
as the pituitary and Hypothalamus which send instructions to the
Thyroid gland to either make or release the hormones.

A Pituitary disorder causes hypothyroidism by failing to produce
enough of Thyroid-Stimulating Hormone (TSH) which tells your
thyroid how much hormone to make.

A Hypothalamus disorder means the brain does not produce enough
Thyroid Releasing Hormone (TRH). So, the thyroid gland does not
release enough thyroid hormone into your bloodstream which causes
hypothyroidism.

The main cause of secondary hypothyroidism are benign tumours on or near the pituitary and hypothalamus glands. Occasionally, damage can be caused by extensive blood loss within the body - this condition is known as "Sheehan Syndrome" and can occur during childbirth. Rarely does an infection or viral illness cause damage to the pituitary gland.

Diagnosing Hypothyroidism

If you suspect you might be hypothyroid, the first battle is to get diagnosed so that you can start on the journey to feel well again.

In my experience of going to doctors with my list of symptoms, they were often quick to point out that as a working mother of three young children, it was to be expected to feel tired, unable to think straight and have headaches.

I agree that to some extent, my symptoms could have been just part of being a parent. However, deep down my gut instinct was telling me something wasn't right. I felt unbalanced.

The exhaustion and fatigue that I felt was worse than what I experienced after having a colicky new born baby that never slept and two other active pre-schoolers. If after reading this book feel your thyroid isn't functioning as it should, these are the tests you need to request.

Diagnosing Hypothyroidism (Too few hormones)

TSH – traditionally this was the test doctors used to diagnose hypothyroidism. Unfortunately for many people their results would come back within range so they were incorrectly told they were not hypothyroid.

This test can only be used for diagnosis if the result comes back high – a high result is indicative of hypothyroidism. A within range result does not mean you do not have hypothyroidism.

It is important to remember that this test is measuring the amount of Thyroid Stimulating Hormone which is produced in your pituitary gland (brain), and not what your thyroid gland is producing. The TSH test is only one part of the puzzle.

Free T3 and Free T4 – This clever test separates our T3 and T4 from the bound (i.e. the ones that are already in use by proteins that carry them around our bodies) and unbound (T3 and T4 that are free for our bodies to use). The results of these tests will show if there is a T4 to T3 conversion issue, or if all your T3 is bounded by proteins that will cause you to suffer from hypothyroid symptoms.

Reverse T3 – This test is measuring the inactive form of T3. Normally, your body would eliminate rT3 quickly and a high result indicates your body is under stress and it will inhibit the conversion of T4 to T3. This is test is useful if your Free T3 is within normal range but you still feel sick. You can experience hypothyroid symptoms because your rT3 is too high.

Thyroid Antibodies – anti-TPO and TgAb (anti-thyroglobulin) a result that is above the normal range is confirmation of the presence of Hashimoto's disease. You don't need to test positive in both tests, one is enough to indicate autoimmune disease.

There are also a small handful of people (10%) who will receive results that are 'normal' or within range who do still have Hashimoto's Disease. There has been some discussion that the disease is dormant in these individuals, but this is still being debated as many are still symptomatic.

If you do receive a negative antibody result, it is a good idea to request a Fine Needle Aspiration (FNA) of your thyroid. By having an FNA, the laboratory can see if you have any "Hurthle Cells" which are present with Hashimoto's Disease.

To diagnose **secondary hypothyroidism** you would expect to see a low TSH blood result, as the Pituitary gland would be failing to produce any Thyroid Stimulating Hormone (TSH), and a low free T4 level.

An MRI will be used to look for any evidence of a tumour in the Pituitary or Hypothalamus Gland. In most cases, the damage to the Pituitary gland is caused by a benign tumour.

Thyroid Condition	TSH	Free T3	Free T4	rT3	TRH	Anti Bodies	Issue is with
Hypothyroid *Primary	High	Low/ Norm	Low	Low	High	Maybe	Thyroid
*Secondary	Norm/ Low	Low/ Norm	Low/ Norm	Low		Maybe	Pituitary Hypotha lamus
Subclinical Hypothyroid	High	Low/ Norm	Low/ Norm				Thyroid
Hashimoto's	Variable	Variable	Variable	Variable	Variable	High	Thyroid
Hyperthyroid	Low	High/ Norm	High/ Norm	High	Low	Maybe	Thyroid
Subclinical Hyperthyroid	Low	Normal	Normal				Thyroid
Graves' Disease	Low	High	High	High	Low		Thyroid

Key to Successfully Treating Hypothyroidism

Now that you have a diagnosis of Hypothyroidism, you have to work with your doctor to develop a treatment plan. The key to successfully treating any hormonal imbalance is to find a doctor that is willing to work with you.

The road to recovery is often long and requires a lot of fine tuning along the way. Your doctor needs to understand that they are a part of your team not the leader.

You are the expert of your body and you need to be in control of your treatment plan.

To treat primary hypothyroidism caused by Hashimoto's Disease, the goal is to bring your thyroid hormone levels up to an optimal level. The options you have for thyroid hormone replacement are synthetic T4, T3 and Natural Desiccated Thyroid.

Synthetic T4 - Solves Half the Problem

The generic name for Synthetic T4 is Levothyroxine. It contains one thyroid hormone, T4.

There are many different brand names for this drug. However, they are all essentially the same. Levothyroxine is the most frequently prescribed drug for hypothyroidism.

For doctors who have prescribed Levothyroxine, the aim is to get your TSH into the normal range. The problem many people are having is that even when they are in the normal range, they still feel unwell.

They are still symptomatic and unhappy on Levothyroxine. Many doctors will start to treat the remaining symptoms with other drugs unrelated to thyroid hormones (anti-depressants, sleeping pills, stimulants).

Some doctors will assess the remaining symptoms and may decide to trial a synthetic T3.

Synthetic T3 – The Life Changer

The generic name for Synthetic T3 is Liothyronine Sodium. It contains one thyroid hormone, T3. The most common brand name is Cytomel.

A good reason to consider adding a synthetic T3 to your T4 treatment plan is if you are still experience fatigue, muscle pain, constipation, weight gain and/or brain fog. One disadvantage to Synthetic T3 medications is that they often 'wear off', meaning you may multi dose throughout the day. For example, you can do this upon waking, early afternoon and late afternoon.

Natural Desiccated Thyroid (NDT) – The Whole Package

Before we had synthetic T4, which was released in the 1960's, doctors were treating their patients with desiccated thyroid taken from pigs! The thyroid gland was removed from the pigs, dried, and crushed so they could be put into a capsule.

The theory behind choosing pig thyroids is that they most closely resemble human thyroids – they also contain four thyroid hormones T4, T3, T2 and T1. The use of Natural Desiccated Thyroid is controversial and often only prescribed by holistic general practitioners.

The argument often given is that NDT is unstable, an antiquated drug and less reliable than Levothyroxine. However Facebook forums, Twitter and millions of thyroid forums have people who switched to NDT and 'got their life back'.

Tricks You Need to Know about Natural Desiccated Thyroid (NDT)

If you make the decision to try Natural Desiccated Thyroid, it is often a lonely journey, with most of the medical profession refusing to acknowledge the advantages of NDT. It is important that you seek out a support group either on Facebook or in another forum.

As a general rule of thumb, you should start low with your starting dose. For example, most start with 1 grain (60-65mg) and raise every 2 weeks by half a grain (30-35mg). The reason why we start low is to allow the T4 to build up in our system as it can take up to 4-6 weeks.

Once you get to the 3 grain mark, it is a good idea to slow your increases down, as most people find they are optimal between 3 to 5 grains. You will know when you are at an optimal dose as you will feel well, and your hypothyroid symptoms will have been eliminated.

When optimal your blood tests should show a below range TSH, which many doctors will find upsetting, free T3 is in the upper quarter of the range, and the free T4 is mid-range.

To make the most of the T3 benefits (mood and energy), most people take two-thirds of their dose in the morning and the rest in the early afternoon. You can take your NDT with food, but not with other medications or coffee and tea.

Occasionally, NDT doesn't work for some people. If this is you, then before switching back to synthetics make sure:

- You check your iron levels
- You check your cortisol levels
- Make sure that you don't spend too long on a dose that is too low

If your iron and cortisol levels are optimal and you haven't spent too long on a low dose, it may be that you have an allergy to one of the fillers.

Contact your compounding clinic and discuss this with them. They may have an alternative filler that they can try for you.

Treating Secondary Hypothyroidism

The treatment options for secondary hypothyroidism are the same in that the goal is to replace the deficient hormone.

However, surgery may be necessary to remove the tumour. If surgery is carried out, it is more than likely that hormone replacement will still be needed.

My Thyroid Nightmare

My mother took me to the doctor at 14 as I had struggled to recover from a simple cold, my glands were still enlarged and I was exhausted.

I was a chubby teenager despite being actively involved in summer and winter sports. Our family doctor requested a full thyroid panel and my thyroid antibodies came back positive.

I was diagnosed as having Hashimoto's Disease. Because my TSH, T3 and T4 were all considered normal and within range, no treatment was required.

We were effectively sent on our way and thought nothing more of it - and here in lies the problem. I wish I knew back then what I know!

My symptoms of difficulty losing weight, fatigue, recurrent infections continued. Occasionally, I would question my doctor about any link these symptoms had to my thyroid. I was told they weren't because my annual thyroid tests were all normal.

It wasn't until the birth of my third child did my thyroid start showing signs of abnormality on blood test results. I lost 10 kilos quite suddenly after her birth, but put it down to being a stressed new mother with three children under the age of three.

As it turned out, it was post-partum thyroiditis and I was in a hyperthyroid state. The doctor told me that the normal progression of this disease was that it would soon turn to a hypothyroid state and eventually end up back at normal.

Over the course of the following 12 months, this is indeed what happened on my blood results. The weight came back as did the fatigue. As a bonus, the post-partum thyroiditis left me with a goitre on the left side of my neck.

It was large enough to make it difficult to turn my neck when reversing in a car.

At this point, my doctor sent me to an endocrine surgeon to have the goitre assessed. I had a Fine Needle Aspiration to determine if there was any sign of thyroid cancer. Thankfully, the result was negative to cancer, but it was decided the goitre was too big and was increasing in size – it had to come out.

I had a Thyroid Lobectomy (left half of my thyroid) and after a short overnight stay, I was discharged.

The recovery was easy enough. My remaining lobe managed to keep all my thyroid levels within normal range so that was the end of that according to my doctor.

I was still symptomatic but at least I didn't have this growth on my neck!

Unfortunately the right lobe became inflamed and started to grow around my wind pipe leaving me with a slight choked feeling. The decision was made to remove the rest of my thyroid. This surgery was longer and not as straightforward as the scar tissue from the previous surgery had gotten in the way.

This time the recovery wasn't as smooth as my parathyroid glands, calcium controllers, had been damaged. I spent two nights in hospital and was discharged with hypocalcaemia which meant I need calcium and vitamin D medications.

My surgeon discharged me with 150mcg of Levothyroxine (T4) and asked me to repeat my TSH, Free T3 and T4 in a month.

It only took a few weeks for me to regret the surgery as I felt so awful. I was dizzy, nauseated, no appetite, insomnia, fatigue, muscle aches, constipated. I couldn't think straight and couldn't get my words out! It was horrendous!

It was at this point I decided I need to try something else. I went to my local doctor and asked about Natural Desiccated Thyroid. She told me that she wouldn't support NDT and didn't even want to discuss it.

I went on a hunt for a new doctor and eventually found a holistic general practitioner in another city that I could Skype for appointments.

She started me on NDT and a variety of other supplements (B12, Zinc, Adrenal Support, & Vitamin D) and slowly we worked our way up to my optimal dose of 180mg of NDT. I take 120mg upon waking and 60 mg after lunch.

Life was finally resembling some form of new normal! One with energy, weight loss, and pretty much symptom-free.

I still find it hard not having support from my local doctor and was often nervous of telling people about the decisions I made about my medications. But for me, it was a Godsend – a life on T4 only was not one I wanted to live!

Hyperthyroid Overview

- The most common cause of hyperthyroidism is Graves' Disease
- Graves' disease is the most common autoimmune disease in the US
- You can be genetically predisposed to this condition
- It is more common in women
- It is more common in those under 40

When a hyperthyroid person visits their doctor, their complaints are often vague. The symptoms are so mild, it is often not that obvious that there is a thyroid issue.

Frequently, the hyperthyroid person leaves the doctor's office after listing their symptoms such as nervousness, irritability, fatigue, weight issues and muscle ache. They're told that they simply need to cut back on the coffee, reduce stress, and exercise regularly.

It is easy to see how hyperthyroidism could be overlooked. If you do have symptoms of hyperthyroidism, you need to have your thyroid fully investigated. In America, as many as 1 in 100 women have this condition, so it's not as rare as you might think.

Causes/Conditions of Thyroid Excess!

Before we get into what causes your body to make too many thyroid hormones, let's do a quick recap on how our thyroid works.

The whole process begins in our brains with our pituitary and hypothalamus glands. It is up to these two glands in the brain to tell the body how much T4 and T3 to release.

So, the hypothalamus tells the pituitary gland to make Thyroid Stimulating Hormone (TSH).

The pituitary gland then releases the TSH into your body. The pituitary gland uses the amount of T4 and T3 in your bloodstream to make a decision on how much TSH to release. If you don't have enough, it will release more TSH - and it will drop if you have too much.

Your thyroid gland uses the amount of TSH to make a decision on how many thyroid hormones to produce.

It's a complex symptom and trouble arises when part of that system fails to work as it should. A hormone imbalance could occur if there is a problem with the pituitary, hypothalamus or the thyroid gland, so it's important to know which gland is causing trouble.

Graves' Disease

The most common cause of hyperthyroidism is an autoimmune disease called **Graves' disease**. In Graves' disease, your immune system decides to create antibodies that tell your thyroid gland to produce too much T4.

We are still not sure what causes your body to attack itself. However, it is widely accepted that there is a genetic component and many scientists suggest there is an environmental component.

Usually, a person with Graves' disease has an enlarged thyroid and complains of irritability, muscle weakness, insomnia, diarrhoea and weight loss. You often hear about a condition called Graves' ophthalmopathy, which can be described best as eye bulging.

Interestingly, this eye condition does not happen in every case despite it being related to Grave's disease.

In fact, there is little agreement among researchers about how frequently this occurs. Some claim it happens in 25% of cases and other state that it's 80%. I have yet to meet anyone with obvious Graves ophthlamopathy.

Toxic Nodular or Multinodular Goitre aka Lumpy Thyroid!

Another less common cause of hyperthyroidism is a toxic nodular (or multinodular) goitre which is basically a nodule (lump!) or multiple nodules (lots of lumps!) in your thyroid. If they grow, this can sometimes cause the thyroid to produce more hormones than needed.

The difficulty with nodules is that not all of them cause an increase in hormone production, and their impact on the thyroid is limited to enlarging it. Unfortunately, we still do not know how to predict which nodules are going to cause an increase in hormone production and those that won't.

Painless and Post-partum Thyroiditis – The added bonus of pregnancy!

This type of thyroiditis which causes hyperthyroidism is painless a temporary phase that can sometimes occur in the post-partum period after a woman delivers a baby.

This is different from the thyroiditis caused by Hashimoto's disease (which results in hypothyroidism). This kind of thyroiditis causes a **slow** destruction of thyroid cells and causes a drop in hormone levels. Thyroiditis that results in hyperthyroidism is when the inflammation in the thyroid causes excess thyroid hormone to leak into your bloodstream due to the **rapid** destruction of thyroid cells.

People who have this rapid destruction of their thyroid often arrive at the doctor's office with symptoms such as anxiety, insomnia, fast heart rate, fatigue, weight loss and irritability. This is called the toxic phase of thyroiditis.

Once all the hormones have leaked into your bloodstream, your hormone levels will start to fall. Most women will find their thyroid gland will return to normal within three months.

Occasionally, some women will become hypothyroid permanently. However, this is uncommon.

Subacute Thyroiditis/De Quervain's Thyroiditis – Temporary Thyroiditis

This form of hyperthyroidism is rare. Typically, the thyroid gland swells rapidly and is very painful and sore. People who this form of thyroiditis feel really unwell and often have a fever. The inflammation generally settles down after 2-3 weeks and your thyroid levels will return to normal.

Diagnosing Hyperthyroidism

If you suspect you might be suffering from hyperthyroidism, it is important to get the right tests done by your doctor so that you are not misdiagnosed. Remember that for the doctor your symptoms might appear to be mild and could be attributed to your lifestyle or a psychological condition.

If you feel that your thyroid gland is bigger than normal, then you need to ask your doctor to check this. Remember that a normal size thyroid isn't detectable by touch.

Your doctor will need to take your pulse, it is likely that it will be elevated. Your reflexes may be quicker than normal. It's possible that if you have Graves' disease, you may have some irregularities with your eyes.

The blood tests you need to request are:

TSH – traditionally, this was the test doctors used to diagnose all thyroid disorders. Unfortunately for many people, their results would come back within range so they were incorrectly told they were not hyperthyroid.

This test can only be used for diagnosis if the result comes back low – a low result is indicative of hyperthyroidism. A within range result does not mean you do not have hyperthyroidism.

It is important to remember that this test is measuring the amount of Thyroid Stimulating Hormone which is produced in your pituitary gland (brain) and not what your thyroid gland is producing. The TSH test is only one part of the puzzle.

Free T3 and Free T4 – This clever test separates our T3 and T4 from the bound (i.e. the ones that are already in use by proteins that carry them around our bodies) and unbound (T3 and T4 that are free for our bodies to use). To confirm hyperthyroidism, you would be looking for high values and above range for your Free T3 and Free T4.

Radioactive Iodine Uptake (Thyroid Scan) – this is test is often used when Graves' disease is suspected. If you are asked to do this test, you will be asked to take a small amount of radioactive iodine (liquid or capsule form).

Over the course of 4-6 hours, this iodine will make its way to your thyroid. At this point, you will have a scan taken and then a follow up scan 24 hours later. Abnormal results could indicate a couple of things.

If your thyroid is enlarged or off centre this could be suggestive of a tumour. If a part of your thyroid appears lighter that is indicative that there is a thyroid problem.

If nodules show darker that points to over activity. Finally they will look at how much iodine has collected in your thyroid, too much iodine means your thyroid is overactive and too little iodine, underactive.

Thyroid Condition	TSH	Free T3	Free T4	rT3	TRH	Anti Bodies	Issue is with
Hypothyroid *Primary	High	Low/ Norm	Low	Low	High	Maybe	Thyroid
*Secondary	Norm/ Low	Low/ Norm	Low/ Norm	Low		Maybe	Pituitary Hypotha lamus
Subclinical Hypothyroid	High	Low/ Norm	Low/ Norm				Thyroid
Hashimoto's	Variable	Variable	Variable	Variable	Variable	High	Thyroid
Hyperthyroid	Low	High/ Norm	High/ Norm	High	Low	Maybe	Thyroid
Subclinical Hyperthyroid	Low	Normal	Normal				Thyroid
Graves' Disease	Low	High	High	High	Low		Thyroid

Unravelling Hyperthyroidism Treatment Options

Treatment is considered simple by most doctors and the first line treatment option is anti-thyroid drugs. There are two commonly prescribed: Carbimazole and Methimazole.

Most people find the Carbimazole itching side effects unbearable, so many opt for Methimzole or Propylthiouracil which have fewer side effects. These drugs work by blocking the thyroid gland's ability to make new thyroid hormone.

Alternatively you could opt for **Radioactive Iodine** (RAI) which destroys the thyroid gland and stops the overproduction of hormones. For most people, one treatment is enough and most are cured from their hyperthyroid state between 3-6 months after the treatment.

Some may need a second or third RAI treatment to destroy enough of the gland to stop the production of hormones. Unfortunately, a side effect of this treatment is that most people end up being hypothyroid.

This could happen two months after treatment or decades after treatment. Another way to stop hyperthyroidism is to opt for thyroid surgery called thyroidectomy.

This is the removal of your thyroid gland. Most people spend 2 days in hospital and require thyroid hormone replacement therapy for rest of their life.

My Thyroid's Funeral Story!

Thyroid surgery is not for the faint hearted! I am currently recovering from thyroid surgery and it wasn't quite what I expected!

The surgery itself went for about 3 hours, and I woke to find a drain stitched into my wound and a lot of yellow antiseptic dye on my neck. The incision is about 7cms long and looks like a smiling face!

When I woke in recovery, the first thing I noticed was how sore my throat was and I felt nauseated. I didn't sleep much that first night and in the morning, I had the drain removed was able to get up and moving.

I had planned on trying to get an early discharge, but the nausea hadn't abated and dizziness had started. After the morning blood tests, we discovered my parathyroid glands had been damaged during the surgery and my calcium levels had dropped below the normal range.

This would explain the weird feeling I was having in my hands! They were tingling, almost like my fingers had goose bumps!

It was a very weird sensation. But within half an hour of taking some strong calcium and vitamin D, this seemed to ease.

The second night, I slept a little more but the pins and needles kept coming back and it was at this point I realised that these calcium levels were going to give me grief.

I was discharged from hospital on day 3 and over the following weeks, I learnt to dose myself with calcium using my symptoms as a guide.

I am hopeful that in the following 6 months, my poor bruised parathyroids will kick into action and I will be able to ditch the calcium. Otherwise, I will be supplementing my thyroid and parathyroid hormones for the rest of my life.

It's not the end of the world but just something else to watch.

The incision and wound healed so quickly. After 2 weeks, it looked like it was an old scar and I had no issues moving my neck. It doesn't hurt or affect me in any way and people are shocked when they hear how recent it was!

Euthyroid Maddness

- Are you borderline hypothyroid?
- Do you have subclinical hypothyroidism or hyperthyroidism?
- Do you have an autoimmune disease that is attacking your thyroid gland?
- Do you have secondary hypothyroidism?

The term Euthyroid is used to describe a normal functioning thyroid gland.

Remembering that most doctors see the TSH test as the gold standard for thyroid testing. If it comes back and it's within the normal range, you will be labelled Euthyroid. The doctor will conclude that your symptoms are not caused by a sick thyroid.

If you have a normal TSH but have hypothyroid symptoms, it is important that your Free T3, Free T4, Reverse T3 and Thyroid Antibodies are tested. If all of these results fall within the normal range, it is important to then assess whether your results are at the higher or lower end of the scale.

If your results are not in the optimal ranges, you need to consider if you are borderline hypothyroid or have subclinical hypothyroidism.

If your results show that you have antibodies (suggesting an autoimmune disease) but your TSH, Free T3, Free T4 and Reverse T3 are within normal range, you are symptomatic. It would be worth pursuing a trial of thyroid medication.

Many patients find that they can slow the disease process down and improve their symptoms by taking thyroid medication before their levels are outside the normal range.

Another disadvantage to looking at a normal TSH result in isolation is that it only tells you that the pituitary is producing TSH. It doesn't tell you about the health of your thyroid.

If the TSH is low, does it mean your thyroid gland is producing an excess of thyroid hormones? Or is your pituitary gland not functioning properly?

The moral of the story is that if you have symptoms, then keep asking your doctor more questions.

Thyroid Cancer

- Thyroid cancer is rare
- Most Thyroid cancer is Papillary which is very treatable
- Thyroid cancer starts in a nodule
- There are very few, if any, symptoms

Thankfully, thyroid cancer is one of the rarer types you could get. Less than 1 in 10 thyroid nodules contain cancer.

For every person diagnosed with thyroid cancer, there are approximately five diagnosed with breast cancer. It is also a very treatable cancer with and the long term outlook for thyroid cancer patients is positive.

Typically thyroid cancer starts in a nodule (lump) and doesn't usually cause any symptoms. A large nodule or lump may cause issues if it compressing the windpipe and can occasionally cause hoarseness of the voice.

It is not possible to diagnose thyroid cancer through blood tests. A nodule or lump has to be tested through a Fine Needle Aspiration or after surgical removal of the thyroid.

There are four main types of thyroid cancer:

Papillary Thyroid Cancer – almost 80% of thyroid cancer are Papillary. This type of cancer grows slowly and spreads to the lymph nodes in your neck. This type of cancer is very treatable and had an excellent outlook.

Follicular Thyroid Cancer – approximately 10% of thyroid cancers are Follicular and more commonly occurs in older patients. Follicular cancer spreads to lymph nodes in the neck and then spreads throughout the body starting with the blood vessels.

Medullary Thyroid Cancer – accounts for 5% of thyroid cancers and seems to run in families and the affected person is likely to have more than one endocrine issue. If a family member has this type of cancer, the rest of the family can be tested to allow early diagnosis and treatment.

Anaplastic Thyroid Cancer – thankfully, the rarest type of thyroid cancer with about 2% of cases being anaplastic. This type of cancer is extremely aggressive and the most people do not respond well to treatment.

There are two options for treating thyroid cancer, the first being surgery and the surgical removal of the thyroid gland. The other is Radioactive Iodine Therapy.

The goal being to either remove the gland or destroy it. These patients will then need to be treated for hypothyroidism as a result of this treatment.

7 Steps to Beating Your Thyroid Fog!

Step 1 – Get your thyroid levels into the optimal zone!

Step 2 – Eat a thyroid friendly diet which is rich in fruits, vegetables, whole grains and lean proteins.

Step 3 – Banish the sugar in your diet!!!!

Step 4 – Swap your caffeine fix for a lovely rehydrating glass of water!

Step 5 – Consciously swap your negative thought patterns with positive ones! The power of positive thought!!!

Step 6 – Go for a walk at least 5 days of the week for 30 minutes!!

Step 7 – Set yourself up for a good sleep each night by practicing good sleep hygiene!

These 7 simples steps will help reduce your thyroid fog and give you more energy each day!!!

Chapter Three:
Adrenal Chaos

"Life is like riding a bicycle. To keep your balance, you must keep moving."– Albert Einstein

- Adrenal Fatigue is not recognised by many mainstream medical practitioners
- Glucocorticoids and mineralocorticoids are steroid hormones
- A one off cortisol test is not sufficient, you to measure 4 points of your day
- An Addisonian Crisis is a life threatening event

Adrenal 101

We have two adrenal glands that are about 1.5 inches in height and 3 inches in length. They sit on top of each of our kidneys. Each of the glands is made up of two parts.

The outer adrenal gland is called the adrenal cortex and the inner is called the adrenal medulla. Each of these two parts produces different hormones and carries out a different task in our body.

The most important difference between these two parts is that the hormones released by the adrenal cortex (outer adrenal gland) are necessary for us to live. The hormones released by the adrenal medulla (inner adrenal gland) are not considered essential.

Adrenal Cortex

The Adrenal Cortex produces corticosteroid hormones - a group of steroid hormones which help our metabolism and deal with inflammation. Within this group of steroid hormones there are two main types - glucocorticoid and mineralocorticoids.

For our adrenal cortex to release glucocorticoids, it needs to receive a message from our hypothalamus, corticotrophin-releasing hormone (CRH), and pituitary glands, adrenal corticotropic hormone (ACTH), in our brain. Our mineralocorticoids rely on our kidneys to tell them what to release.

I am sure you are now wondering what on earth glucocorticoids and mineralocorticoids are.

Glucocorticoids (steroid hormones) released by our adrenal cortex are Hydrocortisone and Corticosterone. **Hydrocortisone** is often called cortisol and its job is to manage how we metabolise fats, proteins and carbohydrates into energy. It also has a role in regulating our blood pressure.

Corticosterone works with Hydrocortisone to ensure our immune system is responding correctly.

The most important **Mineralocorticoids** released by the Adrenal Cortex is **Aldosterone** which is responsible to managing our body's salt and water balance. This salt and water balance is important for blood pressure control.

The adrenal cortex also releases some male and female sex hormones. However, if the ovaries or testes are functioning correctly, the volume produced by the adrenal cortex is overshadowed by what is being produced elsewhere in the bodies.

Adrenal Medulla

Most doctors tell us that the adrenal medulla isn't that important. While we don't need them in the physical life-or-death sense, we do need it to deal with modern day stresses.

The hormones that the inner part of the adrenal glands produce are triggered by our sympathetic nervous system.

So if you were in an accident, your sympathetic nervous system (i.e. the fight or flight response) would kick into gear. It will send a message to your adrenal medulla to release hormones that will help you deal with the stressful event.

The two main hormones released by the Adrenal Medulla are Epinephrine and Norepinephrine.

Epinephrine is more commonly called adrenaline. It's the rush you get when your body is put under stress. Your heart races and all your blood gets pumped to your muscles and brain.

It also sends a message to your liver to spike your blood sugar, giving you all the tools you need to run faster than you have before!

Norepinephrine, otherwise known as noradrenaline, works with epinephrine to bring your body back to a calm state after the stressful event. It specifically narrows your blood vessels and causes high blood pressure.

Symptoms

How do we know if our adrenal glands are unbalanced? A lot can be uncovered by the looking at the symptoms. The following table is a list of common symptoms in patients with adrenal insufficiency or excess.

Remember, if you believe you have 5 or more of the symptoms on either list, it is very suggestive that your adrenal glands are not functioning as they should. If you have 3-4 symptoms on the list, it is still likely that your adrenal glands could be the cause.

If it's less than 3, we can't rule it out and it needs further investigation.

Adrenal Hormone Insufficiency	Adrenal Hormone Excess
Exhausted no matter how much sleep you get	Struggle to get to sleep even though you're tired
Burn Out	Crave sugar particularly after a meal
You use stimulants to stay awake	Carry extra weight around your midsection/abdominals
You feel negative most of the time	Feel bloated
You feel irrational	Eczema, thin skin or other skin conditions
You have bouts of crying over things you wouldn't normally cry over	Feel like your heart is racing
You feel emotionally fragile	High blood pressure
Low blood pressure	Shakiness between meals
You feel dizzy if you stand up from lying down	Reflux

Adrenal Hormone Insufficiency	Adrenal Hormone Excess
Frequent infections or illness	Pink or purple stretch marks on your belly or back
Low blood sugar	Irregular menstrual cycles
Crave salty foods	Often anxious
Nausea	Irritability or just don't feel like yourself
Diarrhoea, constipation or alternate between both	Have trouble falling pregnant
Insomnia and have trouble staying asleep	Crave carbohydrates
Awake in the early hours of the morning	

Adrenal Fatigue vs Adrenal Insufficiency Confusion

One of the most frustrating things about adrenal insufficiency is the controversy around Adrenal Fatigue. The term Adrenal Fatigue became popular when James Wilson, a naturopath and chiropractor, published a book on Adrenal Fatigue in 1998.

Endocrinologists all over the world declared that Adrenal Fatigue was not a real medical condition. These same professionals still maintain the disease does not exist and that the 'real' condition is adrenal insufficiency.

The table below shows the symptoms generally reported for the two conditions.
I may not be a medical professional, but the lists look reasonably similar.

In my opinion, these two are the same condition. It's just that they're on a continuum of severity with untreated adrenal fatigue leading to adrenal insufficiency.

Adrenal Fatigue	Adrenal Insufficiency
Tiredness	Fatigue
Difficulty getting to sleep and waking up	Muscle weakness
Craving salt and/or sugar	Weight loss, lost appetite
Weight Loss	Low blood pressure
The need for stimulants	Depression and irritability
Lightheadedness	Craving for salt
Hair Loss	Headaches
Skin Discolouration	Sweating
	Loss of libido

Causes of Adrenal Insufficiency

- The most common cause of adrenal insufficiency is autoimmune, Addison's Disease
- Nearly everyone with primary adrenal insufficiency suffers from fatigue and weight loss
- To find out if your adrenal insufficiency is primary or secondary, your blood ACTH level has to be measured

There are a few reasons why your body may fail to produce enough cortisol.

It might be because you have a type of adrenal gland disorder (primary adrenal insufficiency). The problem could also be related to the pituitary gland (secondary adrenal insufficiency) which does secrete enough ACTH for your adrenal glands.

Primary Adrenal Insufficiency

Addison's Disease

For 80% of Addison's disease patients, it was an autoimmune condition that caused their immune system to attack the adrenal cortex (outer layer of the adrenal gland) as if it were harmful.

Over time, the disease eventually destroys enough of our adrenal gland to stop it from producing enough cortisol and aldosterone. This is when they start to see symptoms. The rest of Addison's disease patients have one of the following:

- A genetic defect that means the adrenal glands did not develop properly
- An adrenal haemorrhage
- Surgical removal of the adrenal gland
- Amyloidosis (When an abnormal protein called amyloid builds up in your organs)
- Infection
- Cancer

Causes of Secondary Adrenal Insufficiency

Secondary adrenal insufficiency is easily identified because if the pituitary gland is not releasing ACTH. The adrenal glands will produce little cortisol, but the aldosterone will remain at its normal levels.

A common cause of secondary adrenal insufficiency is when a patient who is taking a glucocorticoid hormone (like prednisone for asthma or rheumatoid arthritis) suddenlly stops their medication. Less common causes are tumours in (or near) the pituitary gland, or surgery to remove part (or all) of the pituitary gland.

Diagnosing Adrenal Insufficiency

To diagnose adrenal insufficiency, your doctor needs to test your **cortisol** levels. Unfortunately, a one-off blood cortisol test isn't going to give you enough information.

Thus, it is best if you have 4 samples taken at different times of the day.

Medical professionals who acknowledge the Adrenal Fatigue condition prefer saliva cortisol testing over blood as they believe it is more accurate.

Once you have proven your cortisol is too low, your doctor is likely to request an **ACTH Stimulation** Test. This test is used to diagnose Addison's disease.

Your blood will be drawn before you are given an injection of ACTH followed by a repeated blood test 30 and 60 minutes after the injection of ACTH.

If you have adrenal insufficiency, your levels will either not respond at all, or poorly to the injection. This outcome would be considered abnormal - you would then be subjected to a second (and longer) ACTH stimulation test.

In this test, you will be injected with ACTH and have your blood measured over the next 2-3 days. If you have primary adrenal insufficiency ,your body will not produce any cortisol during this period.

However, if you have secondary adrenal insufficiency, your body will produce cortisol on the 2nd and 3rd day.

Your doctor may request a scan of your pituitary along with other pituitary hormone tests if he/she suspects secondary adrenal insufficiency after the long ACTH test.

Treatment of Adrenal Insufficiency

The main goal of the treatment of adrenal insufficiency or Addison's disease is replacing the hormones that the adrenal glands are not making. The first line of treatment for replacing cortisol is hydrocortisone tablets, and to replace aldosterone we use fludrocortisone acetate.

Hydrocortisone tablets do have a long list of side effects and the one that most people are afraid of is weight gain.

However, the theory is that if your body is deficient in a hormone and you are just replacing it (i.e. not increasing it to above normal levels), then weight gain should not be a problem for you. There are other cortisol alternatives, but they also have similar side effects.

Addisonian Crisis

An Addisonian crisis occurs when the body cannot produce enough cortisol for survival.

Usually, the trigger for an Addisonian Crisis is one of the following:

- A car accident
- An injury leading to physical shock
- Severe dehydration
- Severe infection, such as the flu or a stomach virus

These events place a huge demand on your adrenal glands. If you already have low levels of cortisol, your body will be overwhelmed with the sudden demand for more cortisol. The symptoms of a crisis are:

- Extreme weakness
- Mental confusion
- Darkening of the skin
- Dizziness
- Nausea or abdominal pain
- Vomiting
- Fever
- Sudden pain in the lower back or legs
- Loss of appetite
- Extremely low blood pressure
- Chills
- Skin rashes
- Sweating
- High heart rate
- Loss of consciousness

If you experience a crisis like this, you need to get to a hospital immediately. Without IV hydrocortisone, this could be a life threatening event.

Causes of Adrenal Hyperfunction or Excess

The most common cause of adrenal hyperfunction is Cushing Syndrome.
You are considered to have Cushing syndrome when your cortisol levels are too high. It's usually caused by taking too much corticosteroid medication (i.e. hydrocortisone). However, for some people, their bodies can make too much cortisol.

Symptoms of too much cortisol are:

- A fatty hump between your shoulders
- Weight gain around abdomen, thighs, arms and breasts
- A rounded face (moon face)
- Thin skin that bruises easily
- Acne
- Thicker or more facial/body hair
- Menstrual cycle changes
- Cuts or wounds that heal slowly
- Pink or purple stretch marks on your skin
- High blood pressure
- Bone loss
- Diabetes

Doctors often prescribe corticosteroids to treat diseases that have an inflammatory component such as rheumatoid arthritis, lupus and asthma.

The problem is that often the doses of corticosteroids needed to treat these conditions are higher than the cortisol levels your body would normally produce.

This causes an excess of cortisol in your body which we call **Exogenous Cushing Syndrome.**

If you are not currently taking any corticosteroids and your body produces an excess of cortisol, then we call this **Endogenous Cushing Syndrome.** This is caused by:

- Pituitary gland tumour – releases an excess of ACTH which tells the adrenal glands to make more cortisol. This type of tumour is usually a non-cancerous

- Ectopic ACTH secreting tumour – these are rare but occasionally a tumour may grow somewhere that doesn't usually produce ACTH, as the tumour releases the ACTH it will cause an increase in cortisol production. These tumours could be cancerous.
- Primary Adrenal Gland Disease – a tumour on the adrenal cortex (outer part of the adrenal gland) is usually non-cancerous, but it can cause the overproduction of cortisol.

Diagnosing Adrenal Hyperfunction

To diagnose adrenal hyperfunction, your doctor will need to test your cortisol levels in the same way if they suspected you were suffering from adrenal insufficiency.

Your cortisol will be tested either via blood, urine or saliva tests to determine your cortisol levels throughout the day. If there is concern, your excess cortisol is due to problems with your pituitary gland.

The doctor is likely to request an imaging test such as a CT Scan or MRI.

Treatment of Adrenal Hyperfunction

If your Cushing syndrome has been caused by your corticosteroid medications your doctor will either reduce your corticosteroid medications or swap them for non-corticosteroid medications.

It is important that you don't stop any corticosteroid medications suddenly because you have to give your body time to start making cortisol.

If you have a tumour, this can be surgically removed. Until your body is making sufficient amounts of adrenal hormones, you will need to take some replacement hormone medications.

After surgical intervention, it is hard to know how long it will take for your adrenal glands to start functioning normally. For some, it could be a few months - for others, it may never happen.

If the problem is with your adrenal glands, you could choose to have them removed. However, you will then develop adrenal insufficiency and need to take adrenal hormone replacements.

If surgery isn't an option, you can have Radiation therapy to destroy the tumour. This can be done in a single treatment using Gamma Knife surgery, or over a six-week period.

There are also some medications or drugs that can control excess cortisol production – Ketoconazole, Mitotane and Metyrapone.

Aldosterone Imbalances

Aldosterone is one of the hormones produced by the Adrenal Cortex (outer section of the adrenal glands) and its job is to regulate blood pressure by managing the salt balance in our body with the kidneys.

Too Much Aldosterone – Hyperaldosteronism

Usually, this occurs if there is a non-cancerous (benign) adrenal tumour. The symptoms are high blood pressure, low potassium and abnormal increase of blood volume.

To diagnose hyperaldosteronism, you will have high blood pressure that does not respond to blood pressure medication and a low potassium level.

In primary hyperaldosteronism, your aldosterone level is significantly raised and your renin level is low. If the renin level is normal or high a diagnosis of secondary hyperaldosteronism will be made.

Your doctor may do a 'salt challenge' which is to see what happens to your aldosterone levels after a salt solution is dripped into your bloodstream. If you have hyperaldosteronism, your aldosterone level will not fall as it should compensate for the increased salt.

If a tumour in the adrenal glands is suspected, doctors can measure the amount of aldosterone coming from each of the adrenal glands. If there is more coming from one side, which is suggestive of a tumour on the lower producing side.

Treating Hyperaldosteronism

Hyperaldosteronism can be treated by using medications that stop the effect of aldosterone causing salt and water retention in the kidney. The most commonly used medication is Spironolactone which can cause high blood potassium and low blood salt to block the action of the aldosterone.

However, there are some sex hormone side effects to spironolactone. And an alternative that does not have the same side effects is Eplerenone. If hyperaldosteronism is caused by a tumour these can be surgically removed.

Too Little Aldosterone – Hypoaldosternoism

Low aldosterone occurs with Addison's disease. This is where the adrenal glands stop functioning correctly and occasionally when there is **Aldosterone Synthase Deficiency.**

Aldosterone Synthase Deficiency is a rare genetic condition with similar symptoms to Addison's disease with the exception that they are milder. The enzyme aldosterone synthase is involved in the end of the production process for aldosterone.

Without it, aldosterone is not produced at all, or in very low numbers.

Doctors are more readily testing cortisol levels than aldosterone due to low cortisol being a life threatening issue. The problem is that if you are suffering from any of the following, it could be a low aldosterone level that is causing your symptoms.

Symptoms of Low Aldosterone:

- Fatigue
- Dizziness on standing
- Brain fog
- Low blood pressure – as low as 90/60
- Dehydration
- Palpitations
- Salt cravings

Diagnosing Low Aldosterone

There is a simple test your doctor can run to check your aldosterone level. It is possible for you to have a normal cortisol result and a low aldosterone result.

Treatment for Low Aldosterone

Thankfully, treatment for low aldosterone is simple with the use of Fludrocortisone. The main side effects are headaches and leg swelling, but these are temporary.

If low blood pressure is problematic, then a blood pressure raising medication such as midodrine could be used with fludrocortisone. This combination usually improves energy while reducing dizziness and cognitive slowness.

Adrenal Androgens

Androgens are often considered male hormones. However, women also produce them, but in a much smaller amount.

The most common androgen is testosterone. Dehydroepiandrosterone (DHEA), dehydroepiandrosterone sulphate (DHEAS) and androstenedione are considered pre-androgens as they covert to testosterone.

Adrenal Hyperandrogenism – Androgen Excess

The adrenal glands are responsible for the production of all our DHEA Sulfate and 80% of our bodies DHEA. They also produce 50% of our androstenedione and 25% of our testosterone.

These hormones are known as androgens. An androgen excess can cause acne, hair growth, infertility and the growth of male characteristics in women!

Here are the symptoms of androgen excess:

- Unwanted facial hair
- Acne
- Deepening of voice
- No period
- PCOS

Causes of Adrenal Hyperandrogenism

We know that the following adrenal problems cause the gland to produce an excess of androgens:

- Congenital Adrenal Hyperplasia is a disorder that upsets cortisol production and increase ACTH production. As a result, there is excessive androgen production in the adrenal glands.
- Cushing Syndrome can cause an excess of androgen because of the high levels of cortisol produced.
- Androgen Secreting Tumours
- Hyperprolactinemia

Diagnosing Hyperandrogenism

The difficulty with Hyperandrogenism is idenfitying which gland is creating the excess production of androgens.

In women, the ovaries and adrenal glands are responsible for the production of these hormones. In order to treat the condition effectively, we need to know which gland is malfunctioning.

Your doctor will order a DHEAS test – this test is important because DHEAS (Dehydroepiandrosterone sulphate) is only produced in the adrenal glands. An elevated result tells us that the adrenal gland is responsible for the excess androgens.

To screen for nonclassic Congenital Adrenal Hyperplasia (CAH) your doctor will test 17-Hydroxprogesterone. If there are any enzyme defects this test will be elevated. If this test is elevated the diagnosis will be confirmed with a Synthetic ACTH stimulation test.

Finally, a Dexamethasone suppression test could be used to see if your adrenal glands are the sources of the excess androgens.

This test is a 2 day test where after taking base line DHEAS, Testosterone and cortisol levels the doctors will inject 8 doses of dexamethasone over 48 hours. We know that if your testosterone is supressed more than 40% and DHEAS suppressed more than 60% your adrenals are the cause of the androgen excess.

It is also possible that both your ovaries and adrenals are to blame and if your results show the DHEAS and cortisol and are suppressed and the testosterone 40% suppressed this is likely to be the case. If DHEAS is not supressed then it is possible you have Cushing Syndrome or adrenal cancer.

Treatment

Once it has been confirmed that your excess androgens are caused by your adrenal glands you may be offered a low dose flucocorticoid therapy with dexamethasone.

Adrenal hyperandrogenism responds well to low-dose glucocorticoid therapy with dexamethasone or prednisolone. These agents are used with variable success in women with adrenal hirsutism, CAH, and idiopathic adrenal hyperandrogenism. Glucocorticoids have anti-inflammatory properties and cause profound and varied metabolic effects.

Changes suggesting Cushing disease may develop in patients receiving long-term therapy.

Hypoandrogenism – Low Androgens

Androgen deficiency is women is a controversial subject and there isn't much research on the effects of androgen deficiency on women.

However the symptoms reported are:

- Lethargy
- Loss of muscle mass
- Weakness
- Loss of Libido
- No motivation
- Low mood
- Emotionally fragile

Diagnosing & Treating Hypoandrogenism

There is nearly no literature around diagnosing and treating low androgen levels in women. Even Wikipedia states, "It is recommended that androgen deficiency not be diagnosed in women who are healthy." The reason for this is the controversy around using testosterone for women.

DHEA-S can be measured and for women under 50 with levels of <150 ng/dL pointing towards adrenal glands not producing enough DHEA causing an androgen deficiency. For women over 50 the DHEA-S level of <100 ng/dL suggests androgen deficiency.

To increase androgens you can use DHEA and testosterone. DHEA converts to testosterone so for those nervous of trialling testosterone DHEA could be a safer option. DHEA often improves energy, wellbeing and sexuality.

Testosterone is known to improve low libido for menopausal women and when used at the correct dose there are rarely any side effects. However there are some women who testosterone will not be suitable for.

If you already suffer from severe acne, excessive body hair or blading testosterone is not a good choice for you.

Disease	Symptom	Hormone Imbalance
Cushings	Upper body obesity Thin arms and legs Acne Reddish-blue marks on abdomen or underarm High blood pressure Muscle bone and weakness Moodiness, irritability Depression High blood sugars	Excess Cortisol
Hyper Aldosteron	Low potassium Muscle cramps or spasms Excessive urination Headache Generalised weakness	Excess Aldosterone
Pheochromocytoma	Rapid heart rate Headache Sweating Periodic high/low blood pressure Anxiety/panic attacks Hand tremor Pale skin Blurred vision Weight loss Constipation Abdominal pain High blood sugar Psychiatric disturbances	Excess Adrenaline Excess Noradrenaline

Disease	Symptom	Hormone Imbalance
Addison's Disease	Weight loss Weakness Extreme fatigue Nausea and/or vomiting Low blood pressure Dark skin patches Salt craving Dizzy upon standing Depression	Low Cortisol Low Aldosterone
Congenital adrenal hyperplasia	Acne Irregular menstrual cycle Infertility Excess facial hair Dehydration Low blood pressure Low blood sugar	Low Cortisol
Hypo Aldosterone	Low blood pressure Low sodium Salt craving Fuzzy head Dizzy or lightheaded on standing Palpitations	Low Aldosterone

My Adrenal Story

My diagnosis of Adrenal Fatigue came as a shock to me!

It was part of the tests my holistic doctor ran when I first saw her. At that time, my goal in life was to get a prescription for NDT, so I was surprised to find another hormone issue!

My cortisol levels were just below the normal range. You won't be surprised to learn that the first thing I did was jump on to Google!

I learnt that the first line of treatment was hydrocortisone tablets (which I found a little crazy as I had used hydrocortisone cream for persistent eczema!), and that they had a long list of side effects including the scary weight gain.

The last thing I needed was more weight gain. After discovering the wonder that is NDT, I was sure that there must be an alternative.

Thankfully, I found one. Ironically, it's remarkably similar to NDT in the sense that it's an animal based adrenal glandular product.

So, in my next appointment with my holistic doctor, I spoke to her about it.

She agreed that synthetic treatment of adrenal fatigue was something to be avoided. So, she gave me the green light to try the compounded glandular produce (Thorne Cortex) and told me to supplement with a good adrenal supplement.

This combination worked well for me and I didn't have any side effects from them. The supplement I chose was called Quest Thyrovital – it was supposed to support thyroid and adrenal health and the key ingredient was Ashwagandha.

It made me wonder why there were supplements made to support both glands. I subsequently learnt that hormone imbalances elsewhere in the body puts you under stress, which in turn, taxes the adrenals.

I am still astounded by how one imbalance in the body can trigger a series of effects!

5 Easy Cortisol Reducing Strategies

#1 Relax. Schedule time every day for you to relax. Try meditation, yoga, acupuncture or a remedial massage.

#2 Eat foods that reduce cortisol levels. Dark chocolate, red wine and black tea are high in polyphenols and flavonoids and can reduce cortisol production.

#3 Take Vitamin C, B Vitamins and Magnesium. These vitamins are known the damage caused by cortisol.

#4 Take Cortisol Blockers! Foods high in phosphatidylserine blocks the effects of cortisol on the body. Try mackerel, herring and white beans!

#5 Use an adaptogenic herb. Ashwaghanda and rhodiola rosea are adaptogenic herbs that help your nervous system respond correctly to stress!

If high cortisol is a problem for you I promise these 5 strategies will reduce your cortisol levels and reduce your pesky symptoms!!!

Chapter Four:
Sex Hormone Devastation

*"You know you're in love when you can't fall asleep because reality
is finally better than your dreams."*
– Dr Seuss

- The key to discovering Estrogen Dominance is the ratio
  between progesterone and estrogen
- Too much testosterone can result in PCOS
- Premature (Early) Menopause affects 1 in 50 women before the
  age of 40

An imbalance of sex hormones is a girl's worst nightmare! Side effects
include awful acne that persists long after puberty, mood swings that
make any balanced girl's PMS look like a good day, facial hair and a
swollen tummy!

The problem with sex hormone imbalances is that the symptoms are
more physical. They are painfully obvious and can affect your partner
when they cause issues with your fertility.

I wish I had this knowledge when I was a teenager as treatment is
pretty simple and the side effects are minor.

In this chapter, we are going to look at the imbalances that can occur in
grown women and what we can do about it. So let's start at the
beginning - there are three glands involved in the balancing act of our
sex hormones.

The Hypothalamus and Pituitary Glands and the Ovaries.

The hypothalamus produces a Gonadotropin-releasing hormone (GnRH) which sends a message to the pituitary to release follicle stimulating hormone (FSH) and luteinizing hormone (LH).

The FSH and LH are released into the bloodstream and sent to the ovaries. The FSH and LH are used as a guide for how much estrogen and progesterone to produce.

These hormones are responsible for the development of our bodies and our ability to have children.

The focus in this chapter will be on understanding Estrogen as this is the sex hormone that women produce the most. It is also the cause of most female sex hormone imbalances.

Progesterone, testosterone, LH & FSH and GnRH will be discussed towards the end of the chapter.

Estrogen (Oestrogen)

Estrogen is a term used for a group of estrogenic hormones that are produced in both the male and female bodies. These hormones are needed in our bodies to regulate our growth and development of female sexual characteristics.

When we talk about estrogen, we are referring to a group of hormones: estrone, estradiol and estriol. Of the three, estradiol (Oestradiol) is produced in the highest numbers, so we will focus on this hormone during this chapter.

Estrogen is produced in our adrenal glands, ovaries and fat tissues. However, most of our estradiol is produced in the ovaries in pre-menopausal women. The main job of estradiol is to mature and maintain the female reproductive system.

A boost of estradiol causes an egg to mature for it to be released when the uterus lining has thickened. So, our highest levels of estradiol are found at ovulation and lowest at menstruation.

As we age, these levels drop off. When we hit menopause, our ovaries stop functioning which cause the greatest drop in estradiol.

Estrogen also plays a role in preventing bone loss by working with our calcium, vitamin D and a variety of other hormones and minerals to build our bones. It also triggers the development of breast tissue.

Too Much Estrogen

If your body produces too much estrogen - specifically too much estradiol - this can cause a long list of symptoms. In slightly elevated estradiol levels, you may have acne, constipation, loss of libido and depression.

Really high levels of estradiol can trigger uterine and breast cancer, infertility, weight gain, stroke and heart attacks.

A phrase that is increasing in popularity is **Estrogen Dominance.** Estrogen dominance doesn't necessarily mean you have an exceedingly high level of estrogen. It simply means that your estrogen and progesterone are out of balance.

Progesterone uses cholesterol to make Cortisol, DHEA, testosterone and estrogen. Therefore, if estrogen is higher than progesterone, cortisol, DHEA and testosterone, estrogen dominance could occur.

Symptoms of Estrogen Dominance are:

- Abdominal bloating
- Swollen and/or tender breasts
- Low libido
- Irregular menstrual periods
- Headaches
- Mood swings
- Fibrocystic breasts (lumpy breasts)
- Weight gain
- Hair loss
- Cold hands or feet
- Fatigue
- Trouble sleeping or insomnia
- Forgetful
- Anxiety or irritability
- Difficulty falling pregnant

Why do I have High Estradiol

High estradiol could be caused by an issue with the balance of all your hormones, hormone therapy (HRT), contraceptives, environmental estrogens, obesity or stressful lifestyle.

Alternatively, it could be due to a problem with your ovaries, pituitary or hypothalamus.

Hormonal imbalance generally occurs during perimenopause where estrogen and progesterone levels start dropping off.

Unfortunately, they don't often drop off at the same rate and we often find that progesterone drops off at a faster rate than estrogen. This leaves a woman with low levels of estrogen, but even lower levels of progesterone, causing estrogen dominance.

Sometimes, progesterone drops first and estrogen still remains high, causing a more extreme version of estrogen dominance.

Hormone replacement therapy (HRT) is generally used for women who are experiencing menopausal symptoms or have had their ovaries removed. These drugs can either be estrogen based or an estrogen-progestin combination.

These drugs are synthetic and it has been found that they increase your risk of heart disease, breast cancer, strokes, blood clots and dementia. Furthermore, many women were still symptomatic as they were still estrogen dominant.

Birth control or hormonal contraceptives are similar to HRT in that the problem comes from the content of the contraception.

Most birth control pills are estrogen only which only exacerbates estrogen dominance.

Unfortunately even if you weren't estrogen dominant before taking an estrogen only birth control you can very quickly start having estrogen dominant side effects such as weight gain, mood swings and breast tenderness.

Shocking Truth about Environmental Estrogens!

Environmental estrogens is an area that is becoming increasingly popular as we continue to discover more and more chemical or food additives which contain Xenoestrogens or plant estrogens called Phytoestrogens.

The argument many researchers are using is that xenoestrogens and phytoestrogens mimic the action of estrogen and cause estrogen dominance problems.

Xenoestrogens have been found in:
- Tinned food
- Plastic food wrap
- Deoderants
- Perfume
- Air freshners
- Pain

Phytosestrogens are:
- Soybeans
- Soy milk
- Tofu
- Miso
- Edamames
- Flaxseed products
- Black Cohosh
- Dong Quai

Stressful Lifestyle

We know that stressful situations cause adrenal gland fatigue, which in turn, causes our progesterone levels to drop.

The end result is estrogen dominance which causes anxiety and difficulty sleeping. This puts even more pressure on the adrenal glands and reduces our progesterone even more.

Eventually, this causes the adrenal glands to give up and stop producing cortisol which leads to chronic fatigue as well as sugar and hormonal imbalances.

Glandular Dysfunction

Our glands are very dependent on each other, so an imbalance in one can cause another to go off balance. We see this when an imbalance with the thyroid or adrenal glands causes our estrogen dominance to get even worse.

It is important to understand what the underlying issues are before deciding on how to treat estrogen dominance.

Treating Estrogen Dominance

If progesterone is low, a good way to treat estrogen dominance is to use a progesterone cream. The use of progesterone cream allows progesterone to increase and hopefully, reduce your estrogen dominance.

If you find that progesterone cream doesn't provide symptom relief, consider its tablet form. You have to take a much higher dose to combat the lower absorption rate.

However, those whose bodies struggle to absorb the progesterone cream will have greater success with oral administration.

Many women have success using an estrogen metaboliser to help their bodies process the extra estrogen. The most commonly used supplements are DIM and Myomin.

I use Clinicians Women's Hormone Support purely because it is easy to get as it is made locally.

Low Estrogen or Estrogen deficiency

Low estrogen or low estradiol can cause a wide variety of symptoms, making it difficult to diagnose without a blood test. However, most women complain of:

- Depression
- Fatigue
- Night sweats
- Hot flushes
- Vaginal dryness
- Mood swings
- Headaches
- Low libido

For some people, they simply don't feel right.

Causes of Low Estrogen

Low estrogen could be a sign of menopause when it is expected for estrogen levels to drop and their menstrual cycles to stop. However, there might be other factors involved, such as:

- Ovarian cysts
- Ovarian failure
- Miscarriage
- Childbirth and breast feeding

- An issue with the pituitary gland
- Anorexia or bulimia
- Fertility drugs
- Excessive exercise

Treatment of Low Estrogen – Hypoestrogenism

Once it has been established there is no other cause, the first line of treatment for low estrogen is hormone replacement therapy (HRT).

Diagnosing Estrogen Imbalances

To measure your estrogen levels, your doctor has three tests to choose from: estrone (E1), estradiol (E2) and estriol (E3). Each of these tests can help your doctor make a diagnosis.

However, take note if you are experiencing the following:

- A change to your menstrual cycle
- You are suspicious that you might be going through ovarian failure
- Infertility
- Estrogen deficiency
- Concerned about estrogen producing tumours

If you notice any of the above symptoms, your doctor will need to test your estradiol (E2) and estrone (E1) levels. An increased level of these two estrogens is often seen when there are tumours either in the ovaries or the adrenal glands, as well as hyperthyroidism and cirrhosis.

Estriol (E3) testing is only useful in the event that you are pregnant as decreased levels of E3 can indicate a possible genetic disorder in the baby.

Whew…now that we have dealt with Estrogen, let's talk about the other hormones produced!

Progesterone

Progesterone is part of a group of steroid hormones called progestogens. The corpus luteum develops each cycle from an ovarian follicle.

It also produces most of our progesterone which our bodies need in the second half of our menstrual cycle and during the delicate early stages of pregnancy.

Progesterone is also produced in smaller amounts by the ovaries themselves, the adrenal glands and during pregnancy the placenta.

Excess Progesterone or High Progesterone

High progesterone can cause some issues such as breast tenderness, depression, fatigue and low sex drive. However, there is no serious medical consequences of having too much progesterone.

Progesterone deficiency

Too little progesterone can cause irregular or heavy menstrual bleeding, a miscarriage and early labour. It could also cause fertility issues since our body does not know to release an egg at ovulation without progesterone.

However, the biggest problem with progesterone deficiency is the risk of Estrogen Dominance.

Nicole's Progesterone Success Story

Nicole is one of the amazing people I met on a Facebook forum for Estrogen Dominance and she wanted to share with you her success story!

"I was sick for 15+ years. I had done almost everything there was to do. I looked into diet, exercise, stress management, fermented foods, herbs, homeopathy, many doctors and more.

These are the symptoms I had (in random order):

- Hot flashes
- Night sweats
- Insomnia
- Depression
- Anxiety and panic attacks
- Intense food cravings and binge eating that gave me all the signs of being a full on food addict and needing a 12 step program.
- Headaches
- Crying episodes/mood swings including anger and frustration
- Confusion and brain fog
- Not wanting to leave the house
- Social anxiety
- Inability to get warm at night and often cold hands and feet during day - easily chilled
- Inability to fully empty bladder, especially at night before bed
- Mental faculties and memory loss
- Receding gums
- Joint pain, sometimes immobilizing
- Extreme exhaustion and muscle pain
- Low libido
- Bloating
- Uterus on fire during cycle
- Heavy clots and bleeding for 9+ days

- Endometriosis
- Extreme endo pain in ovaries, groin, legs, back, hip, rectum, and intestines throughout month. I found it was especially high during ovulation, cycle, and bowel movements. the hip pain was so bad at times I was limping
- Endo had gotten so bad it was even protruding my belly button out and was tender to touch and push back in during cycle and ovulation.
- Bed ridden most days before, during, and after my cycle and ovulation...and all symptoms were growing worse.
- Swollen and painful breasts

I am now well! COMPLETELY PAIN FREE, and this is only written on day 65 of my progesterone cream therapy! Most women are not well until day 90 or longer.

I still deal with some pain in my breasts and a few other minor symptoms but those are supposed to take longer to leave...

I am a new person and OFTEN now think...so THIS is how normal people feel. I am the opposite of all those symptoms.

I heard about progesterone therapy being used to treat Estrogen Dominance, so I did my research and found three products. Natpro was out of stock at the time, so I started on Progesta-Care and Progest.

I decided to begin dosing at 200mg b/c I had extreme symptoms. So I was going to split the doses in 1/2 one in the first part of the day, the 2nd dose at the end of the day. (Progesterone levels dip after 1 hours) This is what I did:

- Day one first dose: 100mg (5 pumps of progesta-care) - I felt calm, in a way that I have never experienced before.
- Thirty minutes later I get a headache - added 20mg more, (1 pump) and it left. I added it straight to my temples.

- Throughout the day, I had several other symptoms such as: asthma attack, foggy thinking, suddenly tired, joint pain in my elbow, a general weird feeling all over. All of these new and random symptoms for me. Each time I added on more pump to the area that the symptom was effecting. If I had been using natpro I would have added 1/4 tsp more.
- I ended my very first day with a dose of 320mg
- Day two - I woke with plans to take have the previous days dose (320mg split into two doses). So my first dose was 160mg. It was a better day but still very similar. I has symptoms pop up that made me feel like I needed more cream, each time they disappeared.
- I ended the day at a dosing of 530mg a day, so I knew the next day I would plan for that to be my dosing per day, every day this time out, unless my body continued to have estrogenic flare ups.
- By day nine I was up to 800mg a day and was on progest. I had decided I loved progest more than progesta-care, but was ready for natpro at this point b/c Natpro's concentration of progesterone is so much higher.
- I am now at day 65, at this writing, and have stayed at about 800mg a day of progesterone cream. I'm on Natpro and I take about 2 tsp in the morning, and 2 at night, with one in the afternoon. On days that I need more or are stressful I add more. But I don't go up in my dose anymore. I only add extra to get me through the day."

Nicole's story isn't unusual with thousands of women recommending progesterone cream. I believe that it should be considered as the first line of treatment for anybody with a progesterone deficiency or estrogen dominance.

If any of these symptoms sounds familiar, it is definitely worth going a trial of progesterone cream.

Testosterone

Testosterone, commonly known as a male hormone, is produced by the ovaries and adrenal glands in women albeit at much lower levels that that found in a man. The majority of the testosterone produced in our bodies is done in our ovaries with only a small amount produced in the adrenal glands.

It is considered an androgen which simply means that it stimulates our body to develop male characteristics.

For women, one of its best features is that it enhances our libidos as well as telling our body to make new blood cells. It also ensures that our muscles and bones stay strong after puberty.

Testosterone, once it has converted into dihydrotestosterone (DHEA), also plays a role in the regulation of the release of FSH and LH.

Interestingly, most of the testosterone made in the ovaries coverts into estradiol.

Too Much Testosterone – Polycystic Ovarian Syndrome

For women, high levels of testosterone can cause acne, body and facial hair, balding, muscle bulk and a deeper, masculine voice. It can also raise suspicion of polycystic ovarian syndrome (PCOS) which can lead to infertility.

PCOS is a condition where your ovaries are covered in small cysts. The cysts are not dangerous, but they do cause hormone imbalances, specifically an increase in testosterone.

The main symptoms of PCOS are weight gain, high insulin levels, acne, heavy periods, irregular menstrual cycles, thinning hair on your head and increased growth of body hair.

To diagnose PCOS, your doctor will order blood tests to see if your testosterone levels are high. This would explain your acne, prevent ovulation, facial and body hair growth and balding. Your doctor will also order cholesterol and triglyceride blood tests as these are generally high in women with PCOS.

Finally, an internal ultrasound will be done to see if your ovaries are larger than normal and if there are small cysts on your ovaries.

Unfortunately, treating PCOS is difficult and the focus is generally on reducing symptoms or achieving pregnancy. Infertility caused by high testosterone stops ovulation, so a doctor will try a medicine such as metformin or clomiphene to help you start ovulating.

If you don't wish to get pregnant, then your doctor will try to balance your hormones by using birth control/oral contraceptive pills. These pills often help with the excess hair growth and acne.

If birth control pills aren't successful in dealing with the balding, facial and body hair growth and acne, your doctor may wish to try sprinolactone.

Metformin is a drug used for high insulin levels and more commonly used for diabetic patients. It is thought that the reason why women have high androgen hormones is because their high insulin levels tell the ovaries to make more androgen hormones.

By using metformin, insulin levels are reduced. The ovaries stop producing too many androgen hormones, allowing ovulation to take place.

Clomiphene is an anti-estrogen that has been used to encourage ovulation. This oral medication works by blocking all the estrogen receptors in the hypothalamus.

When this happens, the hypothalamus releases FSH and LH which tell the ovary to ovulate. If this doesn't work, you may need to try injecting FSH and LH to stimulate ovulation.

Too Little Testosterone

For women, the single most commonly reported symptom is lack of libido or reduced sexual desire and mood.

Most women are misdiagnosed as being depressed. Testosterone or Androgen deficiency in women is not well understood since many don't acknowledge it as a condition.

To test for a testosterone deficiency, a free testosterone level of <1.5 pg/mL in women over 50 and <1.0 pg/mL in women under 50 is indicative of a testosterone deficiency.

Given in very small doses, testosterone has shown an increase in symptoms with minimal side effects. However, many doctors are uncomfortable with prescribing it.

Follicle Stimulating Hormone (FSH) and Luteinising Hormone (LH)

Follicle stimulating hormone (FSH) is one of the gonadotrophic hormones. The other is called the luteinising hormone (LH). These hormones are made in the pituitary gland and released into the blood stream to send messages to other glands.

FSH is crucial during puberty and helps the ovaries function. It triggers the growth of follicles in the ovary, and this allows it to release an egg at ovulation.

FSH is also responsible for increasing our estrogen production.

LH is important in assisting FSH to ensure our ovaries are functioning properly. In the first two weeks of a woman's menstrual cycle, our LH hormones need to stimulate the ovarian follicles to produce estradiol.

About half way through the cycle, our LH levels surge so that the ovarian follicle ruptures and releases an egg (i.e. ovulation).

In the second half of the menstrual cycle, our LH hormones send a message to the corpus luteum to produce progesterone.

Gonadotrophin-releasing hormone (GnRH)

The Gonadotrophin-releasing hormone is made in the hypothalamus and sends a message to the pituitary gland to produce luteinising and follicle stimulating hormone.

Demystifying Menopause

In its most basic definition, menopause is when your periods or menstrual bleeding stops. This indicates the absence of ovulation.

Usually, women enter menopause around the age of 50. The general rule of thumb is that if you haven't had a period for six months to a year, then you are likely to be entering menopause.

Symptoms associated with menopause are:

- Hot flashes
- Palpitations
- Decreased libido
- Night sweats
- Weight gain
- Urinary changes

- Mood swings
- Depression
- Anxiety
- Irritability
- Insomnia
- Fatigue

These symptoms can last for anywhere between 12 months to 10 years. Some women won't experience any menopausal symptoms. However, it is thought that about 80% of women do experience symptoms.

There is some literature that states that thinner women are more prone to symptoms than heavier women!

Premature Menopause

Premature menopause is sometimes called ovarian failure. It's when menopause happens before you turn 40.

The biggest difference between menopause and premature menopause is the psychological effects.

For a younger woman, early menopause means she is not ovulating, leaving her infertile. This happens to some women as early as 18 years old.

This can be a problem if they want to have children later in life.

It is estimated that 1 in every 50 women will go through premature menopause before the age of 40, 1 in every 1000 will go through menopause before they turn 30.

While we don't all the reasons why women go through early menopause, some of the known causes are:

- Damage to your ovaries as a result of pelvic surgery, chemotherapy or radiotherapy
- Autoimmune conditions when your immune system attacks the ovary
- Abnormal chromosomes, such as in Turner syndrome (when a woman only has one X chromosome) where the patient experiences premature menopause
- Inherited genes – it seems that a family history of premature menopause increases the chances of future generations going through premature menopause

Hormone Changes during Menopause

At birth, we are provided with our life's entitlement of eggs. By the time we reach 40, this number is significantly reduced and this causes a drop in estrogen and progesterone.

This drop in hormones stops our menstrual periods and no more eggs are released.

Menopause Treatments

If symptoms are debilitating and affect your quality of life, it is worthwhile considering natural hormone supplementation.

Estrogen and progesterone can help balance your hormones and reduce the hot flashes, mood swings, and weight gain while reducing your risk of heart disease that is often associated with menopausal women.

6 Keys to Naturally Treating Menopause

1. Choose GE Free, free range and fresh foods.
2. Ensure you eat a balance of good fats, complex carbohydrates, fruit & vegetables and protein with every meal.
3. Use herbs to combat your symptoms – black cohosh, passionflower, chasteberry, wild yam and ashwagandha.
4. Participate in light exercise on most days of the week. Consider a walk outside in the sunshine or yoga.
5. Remove the negative thought patterns and concentrate on the positive.
6. Concentrate on your emotional wellbeing and make good decision to improve your wellbeing!

Chapter Five:
Obstacles to Wellness

"Only you can control your future." – Dr Seuss

- Sometimes, balancing your hormones is a bit of trial and error
- Remember that once one hormone is unbalanced is has a flow on effect to all your other hormones
- You may be able to survive with normal test results, but you may not feel like you're living until you get optimal results

There are two things that I have battled with during my journey to wellness.

The first was my doctor's heavy reliance on blood results. According to them they were within range despite my symptoms. The second challenge was discovering that by treating one condition, I either discovered a new one or aggravated another.

Optimal vs Normal Debacle

When you have a blood test, your levels will either be low, high or normal and within range. The problem with this is that it compares you to a wide group of people who are all very unique.

At 34, my testosterone and DHEA results might be 'normal' and within range. But is being at the lower end of the range ideal? Is the bottom of the range where you would expect an 80-year-old, and not a 34-year-old?

Treatment decisions should be made based on the information from the blood tests and the symptoms. A low dose trial of DHEA or testosterone could improve a young woman's well-being immensely while still keeping their blood tests results within range.

Each person's optimal range will be different, so that is where you need to take control on of your own health. For every blood test you have, make sure you ask for a copy of your results.

Once you have these, you can start keeping a record of your symptoms at each level. As you try different medications and supplements, or make changes to your diet or lifestyle, you will be able to see how it affects your blood test results.

Thankfully, there are some amazing people in the medical world who are starting to acknowledge that normal ranges don't necessary mean you are fine. Slowly, optimal range guides are starting to make their way onto the Internet.

I have had a look at a few and combined them to get an average for you to use when looking at your own results.

Test	Units	Ref Range	Optimal	Goal
Cortisol (serum/plasma) morning	ug/dl	7-28	10-15	Low to mid range
Cortisol (serum/plasma) afternoon	ug/dl	2-18	6-10	Low to mid range
Cortisol saliva morning	ng/ml	3.7-9.5	10-15	Low to mid range
Cortisol saliva noon	ng/ml	1.2-3.0	10-15	Low to mid range
cortisol saliva evening	ng/ml	0.6-1.9	6-10	Low to mid range
cortisol saliva night	ng/ml	.4-1.0	6-10	Low to mid range

Test	Units	Ref Range	Optimal	Goal
DHEAS (serum)	ug/dL	65-380	200-380	Above midrange
Aldosterone				Above midrange
Estradiol (serum) Day 3	pg/mL	15-350	<80	Upper range
Estradiol (serum) Day 14	pg/mL	15-350	150-350	Upper range
Estradiol (serum) Post menopause	pg/mL	<32	50	Upper range
Progesterone (serum)	ng/ml	Luteal phase 8 to 33	15-33	Goal to reduce estrogen dominance
Progesterone (saliva)	pg/ml	75-270		600 progesterone:1 estrogen
Ratio PG/E2 (blood)		100-500	300-500	Top half of range
Ratio PG/E2 (saliva)		100-500		Top half of range
Free Testosterone (serum)	pg/ml	0-2.2	1.1-2.2	Top half of range
TSH	ug/dl	.35-5.0	1.8-3.0	
Total T4	ug/dl	6-12	5.4-11.5	
Free T4	ng/dL	0.7-1.53	1.0-1.53	Mid range
Free T3	pg/ml	260-480	300-450	Upper range
B12	Ng/L	180-914	500+	Upper range
Vitamin D, D3	ng/ml	32-100	75-90	Mid to high range
Ferritin	ng/ml	15-150	70-90	Mid to upper range
Folate	Ng/ml	140-628	450+	Top third
Magnesium	mg/dL	4.2-6.8	6-6.5	Mid-high range
Potassium	mEq/L	4.0-5.0	4.2	
Zinc	Mcg/mL	.66-1.10	.96-1.10	Top third of range
Iron	Ug/dL	50-170	110-140	Mid to upper ¼
Sodium	mEq/L	136-145	139-142	Mid to upper ¼
Iodine	Umol/L	.2-5.0	2.5	Mid range

How to handle an Unbalanced Endocrine System

When your endocrine system is out of kilter, it is easy to think you simply need to do a blood test and replace your deficiencies or reduce your excess hormones. If it was only that straightforward!

I am going to use my results from about a month after my thyroid lobectomy as an example. I had been feeling tired, weak, dizzy, and nauseous. I also had insomnia and waking up too early in the morning.

I was taking:

- Natural Desiccated Thyroid to replace my now non-existent thyroids
- Adrenal Cortex and Thyrovital supplement for previous adrenal fatigue
- DHEA for wellbeing, libido and sleep
- Low Dose Naltrexone for autoimmune inflammation
- Progesterone cream for estrogen dominance.

Initially, I thought I was taking too much thyroid medication, and it was pushing me into a hyperthyroid state. However, my blood tests showed something quite different!

Results:

	Reference Ranges	Old Results	New Results
Magnesium	0.6-1.2 nmol/L		0.8
Glycated Haemoglobin	20-40 mmol/mol	30	32
FSH	2-25 IU/L	5.1	6.7
Progesterone	1-100 nmol/L	2	11
17b Estradiol	100-1100 pmol/L	550	1151
Testosterone	0.5-2.7 nmol/L	1.4	1.4
Ferritin	20-200 ug/L	72	153
ALT	0-30 U/l	27	43

	Reference Ranges	Old Results	New Results
Sodium	135-145 mmol/L	139	141
Potassium	3.5-5.2 mmol/L	4.2	4.1
Creatinine	45-90 umol/L	66	65
Cortisol 8.30am	250-700 nmol/L	210	269
TSH	0.40-4.00 mIU/L	.18	0.03
Free T4	10-24 pmol/L	17	16
Free T3	2.5-6.0 pmol/L	5.3	7.1
B12	170-600 pmol/L	348	523
Folate	>8.0 nmol/L	26.9	28.3

Since the last test, I had increased my progesterone and DHEA because my progesterone hadn't come up enough. I also increased my NDT after my thyroid surgery since my body was no longer making any thyroid hormones.

What I **expected** to see in these new results was an increase in progesterone and testosterone, a decrease in estradiol, an increase in cortisol and a decrease in TSH. I was surprised to find that while my progesterone had increased, my estradiol had doubled and testosterone stayed the same!

It wasn't quite what I expected and it didn't help the estrogen dominance. My cortisol had increased, but not nearly enough. My thyroid results show too much T3 and a suppressed TSH which I had expected. To find out what was going on, I had to go back to the basics.

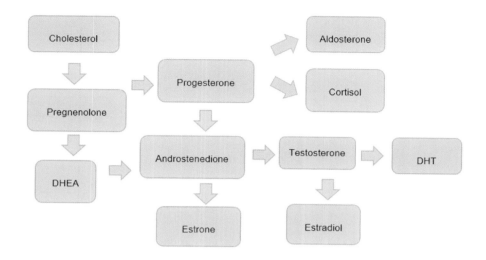

After revisiting the pathways, I think the DHEA I was taking had been converting to estrogen, causing the spike in my levels. So, I needed to stop the DHEA if I was going to get on top of my estrogen dominance.

My progesterone levels have come up considerably after I increased my progesterone cream. The more important result however, is the progesterone to estradiol ratio.

There are a lot of calculators out there, but with a result of 11 to 1151, it isn't too hard to see that estrogen is still very dominant! If you do want to use a calculator, here is one I know of: http://www.endmemo.com/medical/peratio.php

It also looks like my low cortisol levels have been stealing my progesterone to make cortisol, so I really need to sort my cortisol levels and the adrenal fatigue.

Considering I am already taking adrenal cortex and an adrenal supplement, my choices were Hydrocortisone or trying Pregnenolone.

Since increasing my NDT, it looks like my thyroid is showing signs of hyperthyroidism - my body is a little high in T3. After some reflection, I might have increased my NDT too quickly, so I'll drop back to give my body time to adjust.

T3 is processed in the liver, so that explains the high result of my ALT. I think this will fix itself if I just slow down on my NDT increases. The TSH is further suppressed which I expected.

The rest of my results are "normal". However, I think I need to move my magnesium up a bit and B12 looks much better as does my ferritin.

It is interesting that my testosterone has not moved since I started taking DHEA. It looks like estrogen has been stealing all the DHEA and most of the progesterone.

So after looking at these results, I am going to do the following:

- Stop DHEA to reduce estrogen
- Start pregnenlone to increase progesterone and hopefully cortisol
- Consider starting hydrocortisone for cortisol levels
- Add a magnesium supplement
- Slow down my NDT increases to give my liver a rest
- Add an estrogen metaboliser called DIM to eliminate excess estrogen
- Add a low dose of testosterone
- Try progesterone tablets instead of a topical cream just in case my body is having trouble absorbing the cream

You are not alone!

I am part of a couple of Facebook groups that have been a great source of information whenever I want to try something else. The important thing to remember is that we are all different and what might work for one person might not work for another.

It is however, a great place to ask questions and get a variety of answers that you can then research for yourself.

After I received the results above, I asked the following question in the Estrogen Dominance group:

"I have been battling with low cortisol levels for the last 5 months, I am taking Adrenal Cortex (Thorne) and using progesterone cream but it's just not moving up! Has anyone successfully increased cortisol without being on hydrocortisone?"

And here are some of the answers:

- "My energy levels have improved a lot since I developed AF (13 months ago). I didn't take hydrocortisone or other hormones, the only supps I take is multivitamin, c vitamin, zma before sleep, omega 3 and adrenal cortex from thorne. I think what's have helped me the most is sleeping/relaxing a lot when needed, listening to my body and not doing more than I can handle, eating good nutrition, trying to be positive even though it's hard, and patience which maybe is the most important thing, because we have to accept that recovering from AF, especially the later stages, will require a lot of time. Things will get better."
- "Yes. Lots of Liposamal vitamin C and adaptogenic herbs. Its a SLOW process. Understand that taking Adrenal glandulars don't rebuild your adrenals, but allow your adrenals to REST so that they rebuild themselves through proper care including: rest, vitamin C, adaptogenic herbs, and removing the STRESSORS that caused the failure to begin with. Identifying those stressors can be the challenge!"
- "Liposomal C, 1000 mg of Pantethine (B5), a good B complex, fish oil (high grade), Naka`s Threonate Magnesium, and a good probiotic should be included, they help support the brain, body and B5 and C especially for the adrenals."
- "Need minerals, good fats, brazil nuts, wild caught fish, mushrooms, shilajit which is a mineral supplement, and B vitamins."

- "Try whole adrenals before moving to hydrocortisone."
- "I was flatlined and the only thing that worked was solaray adrenal caps."
- "Magnesium and whole food vitamin C regulates cortisol. No ascorbic acid..it does damage to the body! Check the vitamin C you are taking or plan to take. The highest concentration of vitamin C in the body is stored in the adrenal glands. Vitamin C is utilized by the adrenal glands in the production of all of the adrenal hormones, most notably cortisol. Magnesium helps regulate cortisol (too much can lead to anxiety), melatonin (essential for sleep), and blood pressure, and provides the energy to contract and relax the heart and other muscles. Low magnesium levels can lead to symptoms like exhaustion."
- "I had low adrenal cortisol tests for the last few years and nothing worked and I couldn't take adrenal cortex extract. The doc gave me pregnenolone 15mg and 7-Keto DHEA 12.5mg (both very small dose because I couldn't tolerate any higher) and my latest cortisol test after four months was two of the ranges were high normal and two were just a tad high. These two things really helped."

What I love about these groups is that just when you think you have tried everything, someone throws you a lifeline!

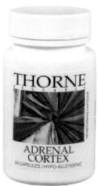

Of course, it might not work for you, but it could also be the key to your success! Looking at these comments, the two I need to investigate are "whole adrenals" and "7-Keto DHEA".

This was the supplement I was taking which is Thorne Adrenal Cortex. It contains pure bovine adrenal glands. The reason why I selected it was because many pepole have had success using it and prefer it to whole glandular products which have adrenaline in them.

The reason why I was trying to stay away from the adrenaline containing products is because too much adrenaline can be a bad thing (i.e. heart palpitations).

For somebody with healthy adrenals who only takes one tablet a day, this wouldn't be a problem. However, I am taking triple the dose to try and stimulate my adrenal glands so I can avoid hydrocortisone.

A triple dose of adrenaline is not going to help matters. So, I think I will stay away from products such as Thorne Cortrex. I know the name is so similar to Thorne Adrenal Cortex, but they are very different products!

Why am I trying to avoid hydrocortisone? Well, I believe my low cortisol levels are a temporary condition. I think that once I deal with my estrogen dominance and thyroid, my adrenals' will improve.

Hydrocortisone is an amazing medication for those with Addisons or severe cortisol problems. It is a life saver, but it isn't an easy drug to use.

You have to understand and listen to your body and dose multiple times in a day. You also need to make sure you stress dose when you're sick or going a stressful time. The reported side effects don't appeal either:

- Osteoporosis
- Glaucoma
- Weight gain and buddha bellies

- Immune supression
- Hypertension
- Diabetes
- Insomnia

A lot of these side effects wouldn't be an issue if you can get your dose right, but it takes time. I am hopeful that my condition is only temporary.

Now, I was taking DHEA and hoped that it would support my adrenal glands. I also thought it would help with weight loss, depression and libido issues.

Unfortunately, it looks like my body has been turning it into estrogen which is exacerbating my estrogen dominance. So, let's take a look at 7-Keto.

7-Keto is a steroid byproduct of DHEA and it doesn't get converted to testosterone or estrogen. It has been advertised as a product to increase metabolism and weight loss (always a good thing for me!).

So it doesn't increase our sex hormones, but it does support the thyroid. It also increases activity, boosts the immune system, enhances memory and slows aging.

Despite my desperate hunting, I can't seem to find any evidence that it supports our adrenals. But I think it might be worth a try, considering the comments in the Facebook forums and the evidence of the positive effects.

Pregnolone is proving to be quite interesting. We know that it is a precursor to all our steroid hormones, but it appears to have minimal anabolic, estrogenic or adrogenic effects.

Apparently, it appears to be effective in enhancing one's memory. It also appears to increase feelings of happiness, promote general well-being and reduce stress induced fatigue. It sounds pretty good and is definitely worth a try.

The Must Have List of Supplements, Vitamins, Minerals for Hormone Balance!

As you can see, I am a big fan of rounding out my synthetic medications with supplements, vitamins and minerals. I found it so confusing trying to figure out what really helps, so I have put together a table for you to use as a guide.

Some of the more popular herbs, minerals and vitamins are:

Thyroid Saviours

- Iodine – which helps the production of thyroid hormone
- Selenium – helps with the conversion of T4 to T3
- Zinc – helps with the conversion of T4 to T3
- Iron – low iron slows the production of thyroid hormones
- Vitamin D – may decrease thyroid antibodies
- Vitamin B12 – for energy

Adrenal Saviours

- B Vitamins – for energy
- Vitamin C – used in the production of cortisol
- Magnesium – for fatigue, depression, muscle ache, insomnia
- Probiotics – for gut health
- Licorice Root – for energy and stimulates hormone production, raises blood pressure
- Ashwagandha – an adaptogenic that supports the adrenals
- Siberian Ginseng – improves cognitive skills and increases energy

- Rhodiola Rosea – increases circulation which increase cortisol production
- Maca Root – helps regulate cortisol and blood sugar

Sex Hormone Saviours

- Fish Oil – helps balance estrogen
- Vitamin D – helps balance estrogen
- B Vitamins – help balance estrogen
- Magnesium – helps regulate cholesterol which converts to sex hormones
- Probiotics – for gut health
- DIM – for estrogen metabolism
- Myomin - inhibits aromatase to reduce estrogen levels
- Zinc – increases progesterone production

Special Mention – Low Dose Naltrexone

I mentioned earlier that I was taking Low Dose Naltrexone. This is another controversial drug that many people describe as a "miracle drug".

In terms of how it could potentially help with hormonal imbalances, it depends on whether or not the problem is caused by an autoimmune disease.

Naltrexone is currently used at doses of around 50mg for people addicted to heroin or opium. It works by blocking opioid receptors in the brain and adrenal glands.

In 1985, Bernard Bihari tried a much smaller dose of naltrexone (3mg) on a HIV patient. The result was that the naltrexone boosted the patient's immune system.

Since then, people have been using Low Dose Naltrexone (LDN) at a dosage of 4.5mg to help gain relief from various cancers and autoimmune diseases.

Overall, there are minimal side effects. However, in my experience, the first two weeks were horrendous. When I described my symptoms on a Facebook page, people said I was "herxing", which is short for Herxheimer Reaction.

For me, it felt like every single bug I ever had came back with a vengeance. The glands around my neck were swollen monsters with a life of their own.

I had headaches, migraines and a general feeling of having the flu for two whole weeks. Then suddenly it all stopped.

I felt great - all my aches and pains disappeared. I slept so deeply and felt so well!

The key to starting Low Dose Naltrexone is to take it slow. For some reason, the dose has to be raised slower for people with Hashimoto's disease compared to any other condition.

For me, I started on a dose of .25ml. I increased by .25ml each week until I got to 4.5ml. Eventually, I scaled back to 3.5ml and this is the optimal dose for me.

It has also been discovered that LDN builds up in your system. To stop any potential side effects, you have skip one dose each week. This prevents it from accumulating in your body.

	Low Cortisol	High Cortisol	Low Prog	Excess Estrogen	Low Estrogen	Excess Androgen	Low Androgen	Low Thyroid	Excess Thyroid
B Vitamins (5,6,12)	Y	Y	Y	Y				Y	
Vitamin C	Y	Y	Y					Y	
Magnesium	Y		Y	Y					Y
Fish Oil		Y				Y		Y	Y
Vitamin D						Y	Y	Y	Y
Probiotics	Y	Y						Y	
Siberian Gineseng	Y							Y	Y
Maca Root	Y		Y					Y	
Liquorice	Y					Y			
Ashwagandha	Y						Y		
Rhodiola Rosea	Y	Y							
Acetyl - L -	Y								Y
Vitex			Y			Y			
Thyme/Oregano			Y		Y				
DIM				Y		Y			
Zinc				Y				Y	
Selenium								Y	Y
Iodine								Y	Y
Tyrosine								Y	Y
Iron	Y								
CoQ10	Y								
D-Ribose	Y								
Magnolia		Y							
Tumeric			Y						
Nettle			Y						
Calcium D				Y					
Chromim						Y			
Alpha Lipoic Acid						Y			
Green Tea						Y			
Black Cohosh					Y				
Damiana					Y				
Evening Primrose					Y				
Boron					Y				
Siberian Rhubarb					Y				
Malaysian Ginseng							Y		
Puncturevine							Y		
Yohimbe							Y		

	Low Cortisol	High Cortisol	Low Prog	Excess Estrogen	Low Estrogen	Excess Androgen	Low Androgen	Low Thyroid	Excess Thyroid
Pine Bark Extract							Y		
L-arginine							Y		
D-aspartic Acid							Y		
Korean Red							Y		
Chrysin							Y		
Saw Palmetto							Y		
Glutathione								Y	
Vitamin A								Y	
Motherwort									Y
Bugleweed									Y
Eleuthero									Y
Glucomannan									Y
Cinnamon						Y			
Chasteberry						Y			

Chapter Six:
Choose a Balanced Lifestyle!!

"Let food be thy medicine and medicine be thy food."
– Hippocrates

- Focus on good sleep habits with the goal of having a minimum of 8 hours each night
- Daily light to moderate exercise is good for hormonal health, while excessive exercising is detrimental
- Do not follow any extreme diets – carbs, fats, protein and vegetables are key to good hormone health
- Cut out the sugar, caffeine and processed food to avoid blood sugar imbalances which stress your adrenals

The journey to perfect health and balance hormones is not just about medications and supplements. It's also about making lifestyle decisions that support your hormones.

I was surprised to discover that many of the diets or fitness trends popular today are detrimental to hormonal health.

The No Gimmick Adrenal Lifestyle

Every website seems to be proclaiming a new Adrenal Fatigue programme. It's so confusing trying to figure out what you should or shouldn't do!

Thankfully, they generally all say the similar thing, so I will break that down for you. This way, you can support your adrenals with a healthy lifestyle including sleep, nutrition and lifestyle choices.

How to Conquer Sleep with Adrenal Fatigue

Unsurprisingly, sleep is crucial in the recovery from adrenal fatigue. The interesting part is that many argue that your adrenal glands do their best repairing between 7AM to 9AM.

So if you can adjust your schedule to be able to sleep through this period, you'll give your adrenals the best chance of recovery.

For most people, 9AM is either the time your boss expects you at work, or the time you need to get the kids to school. So, the best thing you can do is make sure you get a solid 8 hours sleep every night.

Concentrate on your 'sleep hygiene' which doesn't actually mean having clean sheets (although I love clean sheets)! It means setting yourself up before you to go to bed for the best sleep possible.

Try to avoid screens, TV, laptops, tablets and phones for at least an hour before you plan to be in bed.

If you have trouble falling asleep, try taking a magnesium supplement and a light protein snack with a complex carbohydrate. Avoid caffeine in the afternoon and evening as it prevents you from falling asleep.

Adrenal Weight Loss Trick

For those trying to lose weight, the key is not to do too much cardio. Moderate physical activity is the most you should do.

Anything more taxing will drain your adrenals and cause your levels to fall even lower. The perfect exercise would be walking, yoga or weight resistant training like a circuit.

If you have trouble falling asleep, exercising in the evening and can raise cortisol levels which in turn, can help you get a good night's sleep.

Feeding Your Adrenals

The big thing to remember when recovering from adrenal insufficiency is to make sure you have carbohydrates in your diet.

Adopting a low carb or no carb diet will stress your adrenals, so the key is to choose good complex carbohydrates and to eat them moderately.

You need to avoid sugar and caffeine as these may cause your blood sugar levels to skyrocket. Your adrenal glands will have to work hard to level out your blood sugar.

Another trick to keep your blood sugar levels even is to eat regularly and frequently (i.e. every 2-3 hours). Ideally, every meal should have a protein and a healthy fat in it.

You will find you crave salt, which is to be expected with your adrenal glands producing less aldosterone. So liberally add Himalayan Salt to your food.

When you start to feel dizzy, it's a sign that your aldosterone levels are low. It's also trying to send you a message that your blood pressure is low.

You need to include lot of good healthy fats in your diet such as butter, egg yolks, meat and coconut oil. Avoiding fat will compromise your adrenals - as will using too many plant oils such as canola and sunflower.

Avoid high potassium foods such as bananas, especially in the morning. If you consider yourself a bit of a fruit fly, select fruits such as papaya, mango, plums, pears, kiwifruit, apples and cherries. Make sure you get a least 6 servings of vegetables a day.

Keep your water intake up, but don't overdo it. Too much water can cause trouble for the adrenals too.

The Ultimate Adrenal Lifestyle Approach

Analyse the things happening in your life. What are the things that cause you to stress?

Make a list and make a plan to deal with them. Small things like doing the washing or fixing an outdoor tap can be taken care of quickly!

If work or a relationship is causing you to stress, then come up with a plan to start tackling it. This tells yourself that you're actually taking action instead of pointlessly worrying about it.

Take a look at what you have in your environment - is there anything toxic that you could remove? This includes household cleaners or chemicals that could be interfering with your hormones and ultimately contributing to your adrenal fatigue.

Finally, try doing yoga or tai chi to learn relaxation techniques which include breathing and meditation.

Good Honest Thyroid Solution

Eating to support your thyroid is a minefield of foods on the good and bad list!

I will try and break it down for you so you can confidently make decisions on what to eat for your thyroid.

You want to look for **iodine** rich food such as seaweed, seafood, sushi and deep sea fish. They also have the added bonus of vitamin A and zinc.

Selenium rich food is another thyroid healer. Chicken, salmon, tuna, whole unrefined grains, dairy products, garlic and onions are good options.

Reduce goitrogens and thiocyanates which are found in cabbage, cauliflower, brussel sprouts, apples, walnuts, and almonds. These brassica and cyanate foods aggravate the thyroid.

Avoid coffee and any drinks that are chlorinated or fluorinated as they block iodine receptors. Increase omega 3 and 6, but avoid saturated and trans fats.

Reduce the sugar in your diet and deal with those sugar cravings to stop your blood sugar level from spiking.

Try to eat smaller meals more frequently to even out your blood sugar levels, keep your energy up and keep your digestive system happy.

Introduce probiotics to restore the flora of your digestive tract. Good gut health helps the digestion of food, toxins and parasites. Bad gut health can cause food allergies, intolerances and poor absorption.

Perfect Thyroid Exercise

Exercise is known to stimulate thyroid gland secretion and increase your body's sensitivity to these hormones. Try to include some form of exercise every day like walking, swimming, yoga or weight training.

Adopt some meditation and breathing techniques to deal with any stress in your life. While stress doesn't directly affect the thyroid, it can stress out the adrenals which can compromise your thyroid.

The Sex Hormone Leveller

How many times have you heard that oysters are an aphrodisiac? So, the concept that what we eat can influence our hormones is not new. However, did you know how many other things can cause trouble with our sex hormones?

Food for (Sex!) Life

Let's start with the worst offenders and the ones that make our estrogen levels too high!

The Naughty List	The Good List
Processed foods	Whole organic foods
Sugars & fructose	Fresh vegetables
Genetically engineered foods	Fermented foods
Chemical additives	Fish
Alcohol	Red Meat
Unsprouted grains	Organic chicken

Processed foods such as refined carbohydrates are responsible for raising our estrogen levels to unhealthy new heights.

Concentrate on supporting your metabolism. So, stay away from low fat diets, and eat more whole foods.

Balance your meals to keep your blood sugar at a good level. Make sure there is a fat, protein and carbohydrate component in every meal.

Look after your liver and it will get rid of that extra estrogen for you. The liver loves protein and easy-to-digest foods with simple sugars such as honey and dairy products.

Now, let's look at the foods that can increase libido!

- Asparagus – B6, Folate, and Vitamin E
- Avocado – Omega 3 and minerals to help reduce cholesterol
- Chilli – capsaicin which helps release endorphins
- Chocolate – has trypothan (serotonin production)
- Licorice – estrogen and progesterone – increase sexual response
- Shellfish – stimulates testosterone

Lifestyle

Sleep is an important thing to concentrate on when we consider the job that our sex hormones do. These hormones are coordinating a very regular cycle, so it is not surprising that they need us to have a regular sleep cycle.

So, concentrating on getting a good 8 hours sleep each night is going to be beneficial for your sex hormones.

Get into a pattern of regular exercise - it will improve your libido, strengthen your immune system and help with weight loss.

Reduce the toxins in your environment and focus on reducing stress in your life. This way, your body won't have to use precious hormones to deal with your stress responses.

5 Fool Proof Techniques to Rev Up Your Sex Drive!

#1 Destress your life. Proactively deal with the stress in your life. Minimise what you can and put strategies in place so that you can handle the rest!

#2 Connect with your partner. Go on a date!! Schedule quality time together doing something you both enjoy!

#3 Get your sexy back! Do something that makes you feel sexy! Get your hair done, paint your nails, buy a new bra!

#4 Try Peruvian Ginseng. Also called Maca, is a South American root vegetable that is known to increase sex drives!

#5 Check your iron levels. Low iron can destroy your libido!!

These 5 fool proof strategies will have you heading to the bedroom in no time!

Chapter Seven:
The Pancreas-Diabetes
Connection!

"You can, you should, and if you're brave enough to start, you will."
-Stephen King

Diabetes! In the last 20 years Diabetes has been at the forefront of our community's health concerns.

It is really no wonder when you consider that almost 30 million people in the United States have Diabetes. That's 1 person in every 11!

In my family, my mother and brother both have diabetes so understanding diabetes and its relationship with our hormones is close to my heart.

Before we get too carried away let's start at the beginning!

What is Diabetes?

To be diagnosed a diabetic you need to have too much glucose (or sugar) in your bloodstream. For this to happen your pancreas must not be making enough **insulin** for your body.

We get glucose (or sugar) from the carbohydrates we eat and from the secret glucose storage we have in our livers.

We need glucose as it's an essential source of energy for our brains and our bodies! We can't function without it!

You are probably wondering why we are talking about glucose when this whole book has been about hormones but here is the key…

Our pancreas (the gland that sits behind our stomach) release two hormones; glucagon and insulin.

Insulin has two incredibly important jobs. The first is to take the glucose from our blood stream and deliver it to our muscles and fat cells. Once here our bodies can use them for energy.

The other job is to let our body know when we have the right amount of glucose in the body.

To have diabetes, your pancreas can't produce enough of the hormone insulin to keep your sugar levels within the normal range.

Three Types of Diabetes

There are three different types of diabetes!

Type 1 is a condition where your pancreas pretty much doesn't make any insulin! Your immune system has destroyed your pancreas and without any insulin your body can't use any of the glucose in your body for energy.

The insulin/glucose relationship is vital to our health and without our health suffers and you could die. If you had type 1 diabetes you would have to replace your insulin with an insulin injection.

Type 2 diabetes is when your pancreas is still functioning and producing insulin but not enough for your body or your body starts to resist the insulin.

In most cases, the main attributing factor of 'sluggish' insulin production is being overweight. The great thing about this is that if these people were to lose weight their diabetes is likely to be controlled.

If your body has started to resist insulin then you can take a medication that reduces insulin resistance and gives your pancreas a bit of kick start to produce more insulin.

Finally, there is a condition called **gestational diabetes** which is diagnosed when a pregnant woman has high levels of glucose in her blood.

When a woman falls pregnant her insulin needs almost triple and sometimes your body just can't produce enough insulin! Thankfully though this condition is nearly always temporary and disappears after the baby is born.

Diabetes Complications

One of the most devastating things about diabetes is the many complications attributed to the condition.

Diabetes can have a negative impact on your eyes, kidneys, feet, sexual health, skin, mouth, teeth, nerves, heart and thyroid!! It can also increase your susceptibility to infections.

Unfortunately diabetes can damage your eyes and without treatment can cause you to go blind. Thankfully though doctors can successful treat this if caught early and while they might not be able to reverse it they can stop is getting any worse.

Our lovely eyeballs have two parts to them, a front and a back. The front is the part we look out of – the lens. The back of your eyeball is called the retina and is kind of like a projector screen.

To fix the lens (front of your eye) we can use glasses or contact lens but when it comes to fixing the back of your eye it's a bit harder.

With diabetes the blood supply to your retina is damaged and because your retina is a living tissue it will die without a blood supply and you will lose your vision over time.

The most important thing is to make sure you have regular eye checks so that any changes to your vision can be identified and treated.

Your kidneys can suffer with diabetes because one of the hallmarks of diabetes is the damage it does to small blood vessels. Your kidney is made up of many small blood vessels and when they are thickened by diabetes this causes damage.

Your kidney's don't work as well with these larger blood vessels and your body is suddenly not able to get rid of waste products as well as it should.

Over time toxins will build up and you will start to get and feel sicker.

Unfortunately it's not only your kidney's that suffer from the larger, thickened blood vessels! Your poor feet suffer too!

When the blood vessels are all clogged up and the blood supply is limited to the feet, you are prone to developing gangrene.

You will need to take extra care of your feet and make sure you have them checked by a professional regularly so that any changes can be dealt with before it's too late.

For women with diabetes, one of the most frustrating symptoms is vaginitis. Vaginitis is the medical term for inflammation of the vagina. Unfortunately it is more common when you have diabetes but thankfully it can be easily treated so you need to visit the doctor as soon as possible.

The disruption of the blood supply to our skin cells causes diabetics a variety of problems. Thankfully the most common condition is called dermopathy.

Dermopathy looks like light brown, scaly patches which could be oval or circular in shape. You might find them on the front of your legs.

Thankfully they won't hurt and are perfectly harmless and don't need treatment.

If you have been diagnosed as diabetic then you will need to find yourself a friendly dentist! One of the worst parts of diabetes is that it weakens your mouth's germ fighting powers!

This is bad news for our mouths as it means an increase in plaque. On top of that if your blood supply is damaged this could make the gum disease worse.

The complications around nerves is an area of diabetes that still has a lot of unanswered questions!

However we do know that diabetes can cause a variety of nerve damage.

Nerve damage can cause a weakness in your muscles, a loss of feeling and a loss of function that you don't normally have to think about.

The type of symptoms you might feel are prickling, tingling, burning, aching or sharp pain. These sensations mean there is an increase in nerve activity.

Unfortunately the thickening of blood vessels causes major problems with our hearts. Heart disease normally happens when our blood vessels are all clogged up in our heart.

We also know that people with diabetes often have high blood pressure and high cholesterol.

High blood pressure puts an increased strain on the heart which exacerbates the thickening process.

High cholesterol leads to the increase of fatty layers in our blood vessels which causes even more problems.

It is not surprising that diabetes and thyroid conditions have a relationship. Our endocrine system is so intricately linked!

It has been identified that if you have diabetes you have a greater chance of developing a thyroid condition. Thankfully though once diagnosed these can be easily treated.

Healthy Eating for Diabetics

There is a lot of information out about diabetic friendly diets and I am going to quickly give you an overview so you get the basics right!!

First up, it's so important you modify your diet!!

We know without a doubt that blood glucose levels are affected by the type and amount of food we eat. So we need to make simple changes that will make a significant difference to your health.

- Drink only water!
- Eat a minimum of 3 meals per day
- Choose low sugar, low fat and low calorie options
- Eat carbohydrates at each meal but not only a small amount
- Reduce your fat, oil and salt intake

A good guide for what should be on your plate is:

¼ of your plate should be an unrefined carbohydrate

¼ of your plate should be a protein

½ of your plate should be non-starchy vegetables

Chapter Eight:
The Leptin Solution

Leptin is a hormone that is released by our fat cells and its job is to regular our body weight!

The main role leptin plays is to tell our brain that we have enough energy in reserve and stored in our fat cells and that we don't need any more.

So if you have enough energy stored away leptin will tell the brain that you're full – don't eat anymore! If you don't have enough stored away leptin will increase which in turn will tell your brain that you need to eat!

This process goes awry when you try an extreme diet to lose weight! If your diet is extreme enough your body will go into starvation mode. Your body would realise that you didn't have enough energy and to sustain yourself.

Suddenly your body is trying to get you to eat more and build up your stores. It has effectively gone into over drive. You now feel hungrier than ever!!!

Your body is trying to get to you to eat more so that it can generate enough leptin so that you can store some for later.

Leptin Resistance

Occasionally in some people the brain doesn't respond to leptin. This is known as leptin resistance. Their brain doesn't tell them they are full so they keep eating despite the presence of the leptin hormone.

With the increase in energy, comes an increase in fat and the cycle of increasing leptin.

Leptin Deficiency

Leptin deficiency is relatively uncommon however it does exist. If you don't have any leptin in your body your brain gets confused and thinks you are in starvation mode!! It will tell you to consume more and more calories until you are obese and unwell.

Treatment for this is reasonably simple as it is as easy as replacing the hormone with leptin injections which nearly always causes a huge weight loss.

The Leptin Food List!

What is exciting about the research into Leptin is the discovery they have made around the foods that can block and increase it!

Leptin resistance is commonly found in people whose diets are high in energy dense low nutrient foods. So food made with refine flours, sweets and candy, sugar are all detrimental to your hormone health.

Chapter Nine:
The Ghrelin Gremlins

"One cannot think well, love well, sleep well, if one has not dined well." — Virginia Woolf, A Room of One's Own

Ghrelin is another hormone that can cause us to feel hungry!

It is produced and released in a variety of places in our body but the majority of it is controlled by our stomachs!

It has many jobs but the most important one is to act as our hunger hormone to stimulate our appetites so we eat more and store fat.

I am sure in our ancestor's days this was incredibly useful but for some people ghrelin imbalance is the cause of obesity so it's important to consider it when you are having problems with your weight.

Another function ghrelin has is to trigger the release of growth hormones. Growth hormones break down fat tissue and build muscle!

If you can lower your ghrelin hormones you will reduce your hunger and cravings – otherwise known as 'hanger'!!

The normal pattern of ghrelin levels is that they spike just before you need to eat which signals the intense hunger pains in your tummy. Then once you have eaten they will drop off for about three hours.

We know that if we can lower ghrelin levels that we can reduce body fat! Particularly around the abdominal area.

Interestingly carbohydrates and proteins stop the production and release of ghrelin in the blood stream. So next time you feel like your 'hanger' pains are getting the better of you, consider a meal of complex carbohydrates and proteins.

So while ghrelin does not cause obesity, obese people are more sensitive to it.

If you are one of the lucky few who has a lower than average amount of ghrelin then you are likely to have a lower body weight and fat content.

Obese patients who have had gastric bypass surgery noted that their ghrelin levels dropped markedly after the surgery. Researchers believe that this drop in ghrelin levels is the reason why gastric bypass patients have long term success keeping their weight off.

We know that Leptin and Ghrelin are part of the problem for obese people but because our endocrine system is so complex and inter related it is hard to know exactly what we need to change to fix the obesity problem.

Having said that if your weight it a problem for you and you have discovered that you already have a hormone imbalance then it is worthwhile considering your leptin and ghrelin levels.

5 Hunger Busting Foods

When your gremlins are grumbling and you desperately need to eat! Try and choose one of the following!

#1 Eggs
#2 Oats
#3 Legumes
#4 Vegetable Soup
#5 Nuts

You want to try and eat foods high in protein and fibre. Stay away from processed foods and refined carbohydrates as they just simply won't keep you fuller for long.

Make sure you are drinking enough water as thirst can often be confused for hunger!!

Chapter Ten:
The Darkness Hormone

"You know you're in love when you can't fall asleep because reality is finally better than your dreams." — Dr. Seuss

There is another important hormone that we need to consider is the **Darkness Hormone**!! Otherwise known as melatonin.

Melatonin is a hormone that regulates the daily rhythm of our sleep!

For me one of the most critical factors as to how well I survive a day is how rested I feel!!! So melatonin is definitely something worth becoming an expert on.

Melatonin is released from a couple of places in our body but the majority of it comes from our pineal gland.

It is normally released 14 hours before we have to wake up so if you normally wake up at 7am your melatonin will release at 9pm the night before.

We know that about 50% have trouble with our sleep at some point during our lives and release of melatonin is crucial to a good night's sleep.

It also has a role to play with our sex hormones and is reputed to have anti-oxidant effects!

Do you have a sleep problem?

Do you struggle to fall asleep, or keep waking during the night unable to get back to sleep? Or maybe you get up in the morning and feel so tired you just can't believe you have had enough sleep??? If you answer yes to any of these (or possibly even all!) then it's likely you have a melatonin deficiency!

Unfortunately your sleep isn't the only thing that is suffering when you have a melatonin deficiency because we know that melatonin has an anti-oxidant effect and can strengthen your immune system.

A melatonin deficiency is often found in women who suffer from PMS, endometriosis, fibroids, fibrocystic breasts and menstrual problems.

What About Too Much Melatonin?

It can happen! Particularly within countries that have high level of cloud cover. In those countries SAD (seasonal affective disorder) is present in higher rates and so is melatonin excess.

When your circadian rhythm is disrupted your pineal gland can accidentally produce too much melatonin. It's easy to see how confused your pineal gland gets when it relies on the light cycle of the day and night!

Stress can also increase our melatonin secretion as to sugary or processed foods. Stimulants also exacerbate our melatonin secretion.

Should You Try Melatonin?

I first tried melatonin after struggling with insomnia and early morning waking. It was a nightmare!! I was already suffering from fatigue and was exhausted all day only to hop into bed and feel like my body was saying 'just tricking' and lay there all night praying for sleep!!

When I introduced Melatonin I found that within 2 hours I started to yawn and if got myself to bed as soon as the yawning start I would fall asleep within minutes.

It was managed to stop the early waking which is a nice added bonus!

What Does is Actually Do?

Melatonin gets your body ready for sleep.

It lowers your body temperature a bit and starts to make you feel sleepy. It also resets your body clock using the light/dark cycle from the sun.

Other Reported Benefits

I have been watching the research on Melatonin was a lot of interest because when taken in a compounded form it appears to have very few side effects at all!! And trust me when you take as many vitamins, minerals and compounds as me this is most definitely a good thing!!

So What Are They Saying?

The most exciting development I've seen is a trial where they have used a specially made melatonin to treat depression.

I think this is exciting because I believe the link between sleep deprivation and post-natal depression or any form of depression has to be strong!!! My memory of a sick new born and two active toddlers showed a much frazzled and tired mother.

My doctor was so quick to diagnosed depression and dished out anti-depressants like they were candy!

I wonder what would have happened if we had just focussed on the sleep!!

Right another interesting claim is that melatonin acts an antioxidant. This is incredibly useful for those of you (nearly 80%) who suffer from a hormonal imbalance because of autoimmune disease.

Autoimmune disease causes high levels of inflammation in our body and antioxidants help reduce this inflammation!

There are also many articles promising positive link to cancer and migraines but the research here is a little bit sketchy!

The best and proven benefit of melatonin is its ability to allow us to sleep better! So for that and that alone it gets rated as one of the best treatments on the market for me!!

Sleeping Beauty's 5 Step Sleep Plan

Step 1 Embrace your own Body Clock. Plan your day around your natural tendency to be a night owl or early bird.

Step 2 Set your bedroom up for sleep. Ensure you bed is comfortable, the room is dark, invest in ear plugs and remove the TV and all electronic devices.

Step 3 Banish sleeping pills, alcohol and cigarettes! Cigarettes are a stimulant, alcohol leaves you waking unrefreshed and sleeping pills can leave you drowsy the next day.

Step 4 Practice deep breathing and meditation before bed. The goal is to clear your mind.

Step 5 Put your alarm clock out of reach and facing the wall so you can't see the time!

Step 6 Turn the TV off at least one hour before bed.

If you find you still can't get to sleep get up and go and read a book for 30 minutes. Then return to bed and try again.

If you still can't get to sleep and this remains a problem for you then consider trying Melatonin.

Chapter Eleven:
Smile to Survive

"Don't cry because it's over, smile because it happened."
— Dr. Seuss

Frequently on my journey I have become frustrated and negative particularly when progress was slow or when I couldn't do the things I thought I should have been.

Unfortunately this type of negativity is harmful and can get in the way of our achieving our ultimate goal of feeling well again.

The key to overcoming these very normal but negative thoughts is to retrain our brains to think differently.

What we **think** and **do** affects the way we **feel**.

For example, imagine you had tried a variety of herbs to deal with your hot flushes. So far none of them had worked for you and actually some had made it worse!!

A new doctor suggests that you try a new herb that you haven't heard of before.

Because you have already been through this before and the outcome has always been negative you automatically assume that there is no way that this new herb could actually work.

You then might decide to not even try it.

Or if you do try it you set it up to fail by thinking it's a waste of time… maybe you don't take it *exactly* how it was prescribed.

You end up feeling negative regardless of whether the herb was going to work for you or not!

You need to make a conscious decision to stop yourself when you start thinking negatively.

Separate your past experiences or history with the situation and look at the facts. Remembering that our thoughts control what we do and what we do affects our emotions.

"See the positive side, the potential, and make an effort." This very famous quote is from the Dalai Lama and it illustrates how you have to make a choice to be positive. It also identifies that choosing the positive side isn't always the easy option. It takes effort.

To help you learn positivity I have put together a list of the top tips for staying positive!

Top Tips for Positivity!

1. **Smile.** Even when you don't feel like smiling… SMILE!

2. **Rephrase your thoughts.** When they start turning negative take a moment to turn them around and make them positive.

3. **Help Someone.** This positive act will make you feel good!

4. **Accept Responsibility.** Don't play the victim in your own life. These are your decisions and change them if you don't like the situation.

5. **Perfection isn't the Goal.** There is no such thing as a perfect person. You will never be perfect so move on from your mistakes.

6. **Be Grateful.** Even on your darkest days there will be something that you be appreciative of. Challenge yourself to find something to be thankful for each day!

Conclusion

"Remember this: You are an expert of your body."
– Sarah Hackley

By now, you should be feeling much more in control of your health journey. I keep referring to it as a journey because it can take months or even years to find your perfect balance.

Like all journeys, there are times when you are going on along just fine. Then out of nowhere, you get blindsided and stop cold in your tracks.

Just take a moment and go back to basics. Be aware of how you feel and take note of your symptoms.

Your hormones are so intricately interlinked that a slight increase or decrease in one area can trigger a flow of effects to others.

Remember that when your body is under stress, your glands suffer. Listen to your body and work hard to regulate the stress in your life.

Remove stress from your life as much as you can. Find strategies to minimise the stress that you can't get rid of.

Be moderate in your approach to exercise and diets. Remember that for people with hormone balance issues, weight loss will never happen with extreme diets or workouts.

Instead, focus on a diet that is wholesome and full of real food in their natural form.

For some people, synthetic medicines are the best form of treatment. However, just remember that they're not for everyone.

If one form of treatment doesn't work, seek an alternative.

Choose your supplements and vitamins carefully - they are not all created equally. Check dosages, fillers and consider if the brand is reputable.

Never assume that just because your test results are normal, it means that you must be well. You need and should aim for optimal results so that you are symptom free.

Remember, you and you alone are the best judge of your own wellness. Be strong, be brave and keep fighting!

- Ange XX

Printed in Great Britain
by Amazon